PIONEERS IN ANGIOGRAPHY

PIONEERS IN ANGIOGRAPHY

The Portuguese School of Angiography

Edited by
J. A. Veiga-Pires and
Ronald G. Grainger

SPRINGER-SCIENCE+BUSINESS MEDIA, B.V.

PIONEERS IN ANGIOGRAPHY

Originally published by MTP Press Limited in 1982
Softcover reprint of the hardcover 1st edition 1982

ISBN 978-94-017-2676-4 ISBN 978-94-017-2674-0 (eBook)
DOI 10.1007/978-94-017-2674-0

CONTENTS

EDITORIAL INTRODUCTION

The late 1920's was the most innovative and productive period of development in Diagnostic Radiology. This was due to the wonderfully successful research of a group of brilliant Portuguese medical men who developed diagnostic angiography, to the introduction by the young American Moses Swick of the first organic radio-opaque contrast medium, synthesised by Binz and Rath in Berlin, and to Werner Forssmann's heroic catheterisation of his own heart in Berlin in 1929.

The Portuguese school of experimental and clinical investigators was brilliantly led by Egas Moniz, a distinguished politician (Portuguese Foreign Minister and Ambassador to Spain) who abandoned his political career when Salazar established his dictatorial control of Portugal. Moniz then concentrated on his alternative profession for he was also the Inaugural Professor of Neurology and Psychiatry in Lisbon University.

Moniz set his objective to develop cerebral arteriography in order to localise cerebral tumours (to permit their removal by the recently developed intracranial surgery) and to treat neurological disorders by intra-arterial injections. Moniz planned a great many experiments in monkeys, rabbits, dogs and human cadavers in an attempt to discover a safe intra-arterial radiological contrast agent and a suitable technique for clinical cerebral arteriography. His first successful human clinical carotid arteriogram was performed on June 28, 1927 using 25% sodium iodine. He subsequently utilised colloidal thorium dioxide but later discarded it because of its delayed carcinogenic properties, eventually replacing it by the newly developed organic iodine media.

Ironically and tragically, Moniz could not participate in the actual manipulative techniques as his hands were severely crippled by gout, and his assistants, especially Almeida Lima, undertook all the procedures.

The spectacular success of Moniz stimulated his talented clinical colleagues to extend the new arteriographic technique into new territories. Reynaldo dos Santos, Augusto Lamas and J. Pereira Caldas introduced aortography and peripheral arteriography; Lopo de Carvalho, Almeida Lima and Egas Moniz developed pulmonary and cardiac angiography; Hermani Monteiro developed lymphography; Jôao Cid dos Santos (Reynaldo's son) introduced clinical peripheral phlebography, and A. de Sousa Pereira developed abdominal and portal venography. This is a truly remarkable and probably unique record of medical innovation by a small group of brilliant investigators from the Portuguese school, who, within a few years, established an entirely new dimension of vascular and organ imaging. The researchers were as much interested in the therapeutic potential of intra-arterial therapy as in the purely diagnostic aspects of their newly created science.

Although this unique achievement in radiodiagnostic technology and imaging has been well documented in the Portuguese literature, it has not, to the best of our knowledge, been collated and published in the English language. We therefore thought it appropriate to reproduce English translations of the original papers of this brilliant Portuguese team, led by the charismatic and innovative Moniz, whose 1949 Nobel Prize was ironically awarded for his "discovery of prefrontal leucotomy" and not for his more important contributions to angiographic diagnosis.

We have been particularly fortunate in achieving the enthusiastic support of J. Simöes Raposo, Martins da Silva, M.E. Silvestre and others, the Portuguese Society of Radiology and Nuclear Medicine, The Royal College of Surgeons of Edinburgh who graciously allowed publication from their dos Santos collection of radiographs. Introductory commentaries have been kindly provided by Simöes Raposo, Aleu Saldanha, Almeida Lima, Paul C. Bucy, Olle Ollson, and James Bull. Moses Swick has kindly added a note on the introduction of the original organic iodinated intravascular contrast medium — "Uroselectan" — which led to the production of safe angiographic contrast media.

This English publication of the historic Portuguese scientific papers was made possible by the generous support of May & Baker Ltd., Dagenham, Essex, England, and we particularly wish to thank Max Evans and David Oldfield and their staff for their invaluable contributions to the organisation of this project.

Ronald G. Grainger   J. A. Veiga-Pires

Editors

INTRODUCTION TO THE ENGLISH EDITION.

In 1965, during the celebrations of the IV century of Rio de Janeiro, which integrated the First Portuguese-Brazilian Congress of Radiology, the Portuguese Society of Radiology and Nuclear Medicine edited a book entitled "Escola Portuguesa de Angiografia — Os Pioneiros do Método Angiográfico" (The Portuguese School of Angiology — The Pioneers of Angiographic Method). This book was prepared by Prof. Ayres de Sousa, who was then the President of the Society.

In 1977, during the commemorations of the 50th anniversary of the discovery of angiography by Egas Moniz, one of the contemporary Portuguese Senior Radiologists, Dr. Idalio de Oliveira, financed the publication of the second edition of the book, upon which the present English edition is based.

In the interval between the two Portuguese editions, Dr. James Bull suggested the writing of a biography of Egas Moniz, to Dr. J.A. Veiga-Pires, who contacted Prof. Ayres de Sousa to ask him to be a partner in the project. By 1977 Prof. Ayres de Sousa advised Veiga-Pires that the project was not viable, because the documentation available in the Museum Egas Moniz was not yet properly classified and that there was the possibility that one of Moniz disciples, Prof. Miller Guerra, was himself interested in such an enterprise.

As time went by, most of the Portuguese Pioneers of Radiology and some of those involved in this project disappeared.

In 1980, Veiga-Pires and the British Radiologist, Ronald G. Grainger had the idea of publishing an English edition of "The Portuguese School of Angiology" and they were able to secure the collaboration of May & Baker Ltd. for the project. The then President of the Society, Dr. Martins da Silva, gave his enthusiastic agreement, which was confirmed by myself and by the current Secretary of the Society, Dr. M.E. Silvestre. We all felt that an English edition of the book would project still further in the medical world the achievements of the Portuguese School of Angiology.

In this English edition, some corrections and adaptations of the texts and illustrations have been carried out like the inclusion, for didactic purposes, of new reproductions of original angiograms, as well as text-matter thought to be essential, for instance Reynaldo dos Santos "First Communication on Aortography". This last material has been made available by Prof. Antonio Coitom, one of Reynaldo dos Santos disciples. This English edition of the book also contains a commentary by Prof. Olle Olsson, on the implications of the discovery of angiography by the Portuguese Pioneers.

The Portuguese Society of Radiology and Nuclear Medicine is grateful to Mr. Max Evans of May & Baker Ltd. for his administrative help and to Drs. J.A. Veiga-Pires and Ronald G. Grainger, who took it upon themselves to prepare the edition and to revise the texts that constitute this book.

Lisbon, June 5th 1981

J. Simões Raposo

EARLY ARTERIOGRAPHY IN THE U.K.

Although a few carotid arteriograms were performed in the U.K. fairly shortly after Moniz's discovery in 1927, the number could probably be counted on both hands. Meanwhile in Portugal (the home), Spain and Germany in particular, the method became popular for the diagnosis of intracranial masses. In England the investigation was usually in the hands of the neurologist who, on clinical grounds, instructed the surgeon (there were very few pure neurosurgeons before the second World War) where to make his flap. Ventriculography was occasionally employed and there was only one radiologist in England who could use it usefully, and that was Edward Wing Twining of Manchester. I have often wondered why Moniz's method was resisted in the U.K. I think perhaps what inhibited it was the fact that he always injected the right and left sides, and after a very few percutaneous attempts early on, reverted to the cut down method. This meant bilateral permanent scars on the front of the neck. A woman with any pretensions to beauty would resist this, particularly if the examination proved negative.

A minor point which might have made a few well informed surgeons rather frightened was the amount of radiation their fingers and hands would be getting.

The whole picture changed when Kristianson and Engeset attempted the percutaneous method in the middle of World War II. Kristianson performed the punctures and Engeset the radiology.

They were not the first to practise the percutaneous method. Moniz had used it for his first few cases then abandoned it. In 1936 Loman and Myerson in the U.S.A. described 30 cases in the American Journal of Roentgenology. In their paper they only showed lateral angiograms of rather poor quality and they used thorotrast. For some unexplained reason they abandoned the method.

The Norwegians made two great advances. Firstly they abandoned the use of the radioactive contrast substance, thorotrast, which also became fixed in the tissues, particularly the liver and spleen. Up till then it had been used almost universally as an arterial contrast substance. Instead they used perabrodil which was not radioactive and was excreted by the kidneys. Secondly they pursued the percutaneous method.

In 1944 Engeset published his monograph on the subject. Being wartime, and Norway being occupied by the Germans, the information reached no further than Sweden. It is of some interest that in Engeset's bibliography the papers quoted are nearly all in German, rather confirming the view I stated earlier that the German school took up cerebral angiography to a greater degree than elsewhere.

In Stockholm Lysholm, the radiologist and Olivecrona, the neurosurgeon, immediately saw the potential. Lysholm's first assistant, Erik Lindgren, went to work in their famous Röntgen Department in the Serafimer Hospital, and with the aid of Georg Fredzell, a young engineer in the Schönander firm, an apparatus was set up. It was incorporated in Lysholm's well known skull table. A vertical box containing three cassettes was placed at the side of the patient's supine head and a smaller box of two cassettes placed behind his head for the A.P. films. A simple, but very effective, linen band was placed round the head to restrain it from movement. Lindgren, well known for his skill with his hands, amongst his many other attributes, soon learnt the percutaneous technique, and carotid angiography immediately became an established procedure in the Serafimer Hospital. This was towards the end of World War II.

I had spent a year with Lysholm (1938-1939) where I saw about 2 carotid arteriograms — perhaps 3 in twelve months. My first professional task on returning from the Far East after the war was to rub off the rust in Stockholm and my wife and I took the first civilian boat sailing for Sweden. I found that neuroradiology at the Serafimer Hospital had changed dramatically. Three or four percutaneous carotid arteriograms were being performed daily by Lindgren, or by then, some by Sjögren.

In autumn 1946 hundreds of cases had been examined angiographically and Lysholm instructed one of his assistants, Wickbom, to analyse the angiographic features of the tumours examined. Three hundred and seventy six tumour cases had been collected. In 1948 Wickbom's thesis on this material was published in two parts;

(1) the normal angiographic anatomy of the carotid tree and (2) a classification of the tumours. This represented an enormous advance in neuroradiology. As far as I am aware this monograph was far and away the biggest contribution to the literature of carotid angiography since Moniz's work about twenty years previously.

Thus percutaneous angiography had become established practice with the aid of an iodine containing water soluble contrast medium.

So it was that I was able to bring the technique, together with femoral angiography, to England.

What was most important from the patient's and radiologist's point of view was Lindgren's setting of the example that the whole procedure should be carried out by the neuroradiologist. This, of course he applied equally to other practical measures such as encephalography and myelography. He demonstrated by his example that not only did the patient suffer less by being attended by an experienced neuroradiologist rather than a neurosurgical house surgeon (as happened in many countries), but also the quality of the radiography, the proper protective measures against radiation and the technique in general, were infinitely superior in Lindgren's hands than elswhere. In my opinion the Lysholm — Lindgren school outshone all others by a long way at that time. In some medically advanced countries it took a generation before the practical procedures got into the control of the neuroradiologist.

Shortly after Wickbom's thesis a young cardiologist in Lund named Radner had been catheterising the radial artery by a cut-down method with the object of performing cardiac angiography. By accident he found that his catheter, in its retrograde course, often passed from the subclavian artery into the vertebral rather than continuing into the innominate. This happened so often that he decided to take advantage of it; thus he began his work on vertebral angiography and published his thesis in 1951 when I had the privilege of acting as his first opponent (ie. examining him).

The urge for serial angiography was developing in the late nineteen forties. This was being attacked in two ways (1) by continuous roll film and (2) cut film. Quite good success was achieved using the former method in the United States with the Fairchild Camera. This had been used for photographic aerial reconnaisance in World War II and was modified for radiography. It took pictures of an ideal size (10″ x 10″) for cerebral angiography and good results were obtained with it.

Meanwhile in the Schönander factory in Stockholm, Georg Fredzell was busy designing an apparatus taking cut film. As early as 1950 he produced a rapid serial device for angiocardiography taking films at 0.08 sec., intervals. Meanwhile in 1952 he presented his famous A.O.T. changer for cerebral angiography which would take up to six pictures per second or any lesser required speed, up to a total of 30 films.

Dr. James W.D. Bull
London, August 1981

EARLY ARTERIOGRAPHY IN SWEDEN

The vascular system is a basic part of the organism. Lesions in the vascular system are common and of great importance for diagnosis and therapy. The vascular system is an integral part of every organ system and is involved, often very characteristically, in many diseases. These simple facts make a roentgenological study of the vascular system extremely important.

My own interest in angiography arose from my wish to demonstrate direct radiological evidence of the nature of expansile lesions in the kidney, for both intravenous and retrograde urography provide only indirect signs of the nature of these lesions. As soon as possible after the war had ended in 1945, I went with Professor Einar Ljunggren of Copenhagen for my first visit to Lisbon (in 1946). There I met the wonderful Professor Reynaldo dos Santos and his collaborators and we had excellent discussions about abdominal angiography. I immediately saw the possibilities and on my return to Sweden I introduced angiographic procedures in our department.

World medicine owes a great debt of gratitude to Portuguese medicine for offering the possibility of performing all types of angiography. The names Egas Moniz (Nobel Prize winner in 1949) and Reynaldo dos Santos are leading lights in the enormous and important progress of this specialized part of diagnostic radiology.

New methods have replaced angiography for certain diagnostic problems to some extent today. However, angiography still retains it great importance, demonstrated by the help angiographic procedures can offer in therapy: selective injection of cytostatic drugs, selective approach to bleeding vessels and selective treatment of arterial stenosis etc.

For many years past and for many years to come, World Radiology will pay its deep respect to the great Portuguese pioneers, monumental figureheads in our important speciality, diagnostic Radiology.

Olle Olsson
Lund, July 1981 Sweden.

THE INFLUENCE OF MONIZ ON NEUROLOGY

Neurological surgery is indebted to many people for its development and progress . Not all of these were surgeons. One of the most outstanding of this latter group was Egas Moniz, a distinguished Portuguese neurologist. In addition to an extensive understanding of the nervous system and its diseases, he possessed an exceptionally keen, enquiring mind and neurosurgery will be forever in his debt for his revolutionary discovery and development of cerebral angiography. This he did in collaboration with his close friend and professional associate, Professor Almeida Lima. Professor Almeida Lima was at that time a neurosurgeon. Since then he has become the successor of Egas Moniz as Professor of Neurology in Lisbon and is now restricting his activities largely to the non-surgical aspects of neurology.

In addition to inventing cerebral angiography, Egas Moniz conceived the idea of frontal lobotomy for the treatment of certain psychiatric disorders. In this he was stimulated by the experimental studies of Fulton and Jacobsen[1] on the results of destructive lesions of the frontal lobes in apes. The fundamental contribution of Egas Moniz, and the aspect of frontal lobotomy responsible for much of past and present antagonism of some psychiatrists and psychologists to "psychosurgery" was the irrefutable establishment of the organic nature of certain psychological and behavioural disorders.

Paul C. Bucy.
Editor Surgical Neurology.

1) C.F. Jacobsen. Functions of frontal association areas in primates. Arch. N. & P. 1935, 33:558-560.

THE PORTUGUESE SCHOOL OF ANGIOGRAPHY

Aleu Saldanha

Professor of the Department of Radiology, Faculty of Medicine, Lisbon.

When man reaches a certain intellectual plane, he feels the need to strive for perfection and his spirit is moved to a greater or lesser extent to improve his circumstances and his culture. Whatever field of knowledge is his calling, the scientist at first grasps the established ideas and facts but he soon becomes painfully aware of his limitations as far as crossing the great unknown frontiers is concerned. Restlessness and an eagerness to cross these frontiers form the basis of the spirit of the research worker.

In 1924, when we first embarked on the study of medical radiology, the frontier was nearby and long because there were no well established guide-lines which merely needed improvement and amplification, as were available in the other branches of medicine. Our generation had to open and clear the road and devise new methods and ideas on which the speciality could be built.

For a while, during the first few decades of this century, there were few supporters and many critics. It was a period in which pioneers fought on in difficulty and danger but their enthusiasm and their vision of what X-rays could offer medicine was victorious. As the years passed, the progress of radiology accelerated and today it is very rapid. This advance has called for technical progress and physicists, chemists, engineers and industrialists have responded with extraordinary achievements. These have been very effective in bringing about the wonderful investigative tool which is at our disposal today.

Not only radiologists but also clinicians now appreciate the ability of radiological techniques to resolve many of their professional problems.

This ability and the diversity of the problems have had a profound influence on the direction of research in radiology. In some countries this has taken many paths but in others there have been special reasons why research has very largely followed a single road.

This has been the case in Portugal where many investigators from diverse cultural centres contrived to unite their skills in a wide range of topics within the same subject and to establish a real and well defined school, the Portuguese School of Angiography.

There have been thousands of works about angiography published throughout the world, there have been many technical improvements and there has been a large number of valuable results achieved, but there have been very few which have not had their basis in the Portuguese School which is able to cover nearly all, if not the whole, of the enormous field of vascular visualisation.

There are two basic reasons for the harmony and unity of the school and the conjunction of undertakings which gives the appearance of being planned. The first is the spirit of the man, Egas Moniz, who was brilliant and influential and who excited the admiration of those around him by the success of his investigations, and the second is the universal nature of the vascular system in human physiology.

When he had finished his "magnum opus" on the problem of localising cerebral tumours, the Master quickly concentrated his insatiable desire for research on an exhaustive investigation of the many aspects of cerebral circulation. The work of Egas Moniz between 1927 and 1935 came to have world-wide influence. However much we may deplore the fact that the voice of a small country is not widely heard, we must take pleasure now that he has made it possible for Portuguese research workers to cover the topic very thoroughly in numerous publications.

As his modest collaborator, I had the honour to present for the first time at an International Congress of Radiology in Paris in 1931, the first results of arterial encephalography. Today I am unable to suppress a smile at the lack of enthusiasm with which this was greeted.

At that period in radiology, vessels had been rendered opaque post-mortem and there had been attempts to visualize them in life but the execution of cerebral angiography, with positive results and with the information it provided about anatomy, physiology and morbid anatomy, clearly opened the enormous field of arterial visualisation to radiology.

In addition to all the abilities which he brought to the thoughtful and vigorous pursuit of his discoveries, Egas Moniz had the other qualities of a great team captain. With his kindness, his good manners and his tact, he was able to inspire his colleagues, pay attention to them, accept some opinions and give them their proper credit.

Almeida Lima should be mentioned above all, for he is well known for continuing the good work both as a teacher and a research worker.

We recall that Egas Moniz wrote in his "Secrets of a Scientific Investigator" of "recognising his (Lima's) qualities" and "I called to ask for his assistance" and "he wanted to inject the internal carotid". Later on we find "Almeida Lima carried most of the burden when we were striving to achieve cerebral angiography".

It was at the historic conference in the faculty of Medicine in

Lisbon where Egas Moniz first presented his work, that another shining light of Portuguese medicine, Reynaldo dos Santos, at once realised the great possibilities which the research had unfolded and suggested that the Master should pursue his research in the field of the peripheral arteries. There is no need to exaggerate the success achieved by the work of Reynaldo dos Santos with Augusto Lamas and J. Pereira Caldas as his colleagues. Their technique elucidated several of the circulatory problems of the abdominal organs and gave rise to effective surgical procedures for many disorders. Work on this topic is still being carried out in many countries and all the possibilities are far from being exhausted. In the wake of Reynaldo dos Santos came his son J. Cid dos Santos in the venous field. He completely mastered phlebographic techniques, published his well-known works and continues to perform remarkable work in the Department of Clinical Surgery.

Although the Lisbon School has been interested in the investigation of blood vessels, there was a large vascular field in which no work had been carried out and in which research was lacking. In the Faculty of Medicine at Oporto, Hernani Monteiro, Alvaro Rodrigues, A. de Sousa Pereira and Roberto de Carvalho started work on the visualisation of lymphatics and in this field they were certainly pioneers. They achieved the first images of lymph nodes and lymphatic vessels either by direct injection into the nodes or indirectly and their efforts were crowned with success.

The investigative spirit of Egas Moniz could not rest. Along with Lopo de Carvalho and Almeida Lima, he had the idea of injecting contrast medium into the human heart through a radio-opaque Forssmann catheter. The execution of this form of angiography was a notable achievement in medicine and was later to revolutionise cardiology.

Pulmonary angiography, the objective of the technique, was achieved. Contrast medium was inserted into the pulmonary vessels but not to the desired extent, simply because it was impossible to inject a sufficient quantity of sodium iodide, even at 120%, to avoid it becoming too diluted. This was also the only reason why the authors were unable to outline the cavities of the heart, as they had been able to do experimentally in rabbits.

It was seven years later, when improved contrast media became available, that angiocardiography was carried out in man and thus Egas Moniz, Lopo de Carvalho and Almeida Lima did not get the credit for being the originators of this technique.

While carrying out injections into the carotid, Egas Moniz noticed that when there was an extravasation of the fluid, it returned again into the vessels. He honoured me by placing me in charge of an investigation in which we attempted to render the perivascular tissues opaque. After experimental work on the sheaths in cadavers in dogs and eventually "in vivo", we found that although we could visualise the sheaths, this was of only limited usefulness in investigations of the mediastinum. However, the work we had carried out in obedience to the Master's suggestion served us very well in that we learned a good deal about the anatomy and in particular we formed ideas about fascial systems which enabled us to carry out our later work on the radiology of the interstices.

It was this same environment in which interest was focused on angiography that prompted the enthusiastic research worker Sousa Pereira to inject contrast medium in a radiological investigation of the portal vein. He presented the first results of direct, operative injection into one of the tributaries of the portal vein in 1949 and later, in 1951, of transparietal injection into a vein at the hilum of the spleen. In the field of portal venography, he preceded Abbeatici and Campi who by injecting into the spleen certainly improved the radiology of the splenic and portal veins and made it an easier and more efficient technique.

During the development of the technique of cerebral angiography, Egas Moniz was concerned at first with the morphology of the cerebral arteries. The technique of injecting into the common carotid without previous ligation made the examination more physiological in nature and allowed the cerebral haemodynamics to be studied. The blood supply to the brain, meninges and soft tissues around the cranium could be distinguished and the rate at which blood passed through the different organs and parts of the human body was shown to vary. It was clear, however, that the exact speed of blood could not be measured by angiographic techniques.

The problem was brilliantly resolved by N. Ayres de Sousa who conceived the entirely original idea of angiokymography. The possibility, which his technique offered, of noting precisely the starting time and the time at which any given vessel, artery or vein, became opaque was a real advance in the visualisation of vessels. He was able to study the pulmonary circulation time and to tackle other haemodynamic problems in the central and peripheral circulations thereby opening broad vistas in the investigation of the physiology and physiopathology of the circulation of blood.

In addition to angiokymography, Ayres de Sousa made a major contribution to the Portuguese School of Angiography by his remarkable and well-known work on microangiography. Only vessels of a certain calibre can be examined by conventional angiography and there are very complex, microscopic vascular structures and study of these by contrast histography is more rewarding in terms of detail and inference than many other histological techniques. His work has clarified many of the difficult problems associated with the details of circulation in the tissues. There is always an interstitial space between the cells and the vessels which carry essential factors to the sites of their biological functions. Taken together these spaces comprise a continuous system which extends throughout the human body. We owe our knowledge of this and its demonstration, as I said, to Egas Moniz' studies on vascular sheaths. It is the currents in this anatomical substrate or system of interstitial fluid, (Claude Bernard's "milieu interieur"), which carry the nutrients to the cell walls and which take the products of catabolism to the venous capillaries. We refer to this system as the plasma-tissue circulation and it is distinct from the circulation of blood or lymph; we are attempting to study its morphology and physiology by rendering it opaque. I consider that visualisation of the plasma-tissue circulation is at the extreme limit of angiography.

I have described this chain of research workers, some important and some of lesser significance, in order to give an idea of the overall background and nature of the Portuguese School of Angiography.

Over about 40 years of professional activity, I have seen ample evidence of the progress of radiology in our country. The matters I have described have not inhibited research but clinicians and radiologists have been faced with many problems and an enormous amount of work has been carried out. Without an official research organisation, which some countries are just beginning to establish, the effort in the fight against numerous deficiencies would be expended largely by individuals and it could rely only on the dedication, enthusiasm and spirit of self-sacrifice of the research workers.

I confidently expect that the new generation will have better conditions in which to achieve the fulfilment of their scientific ambitions. However, even if the circumstances are not ideal, our spirits should be lifted by remembering the example of Egas Moniz who achieved so much with so few resources.

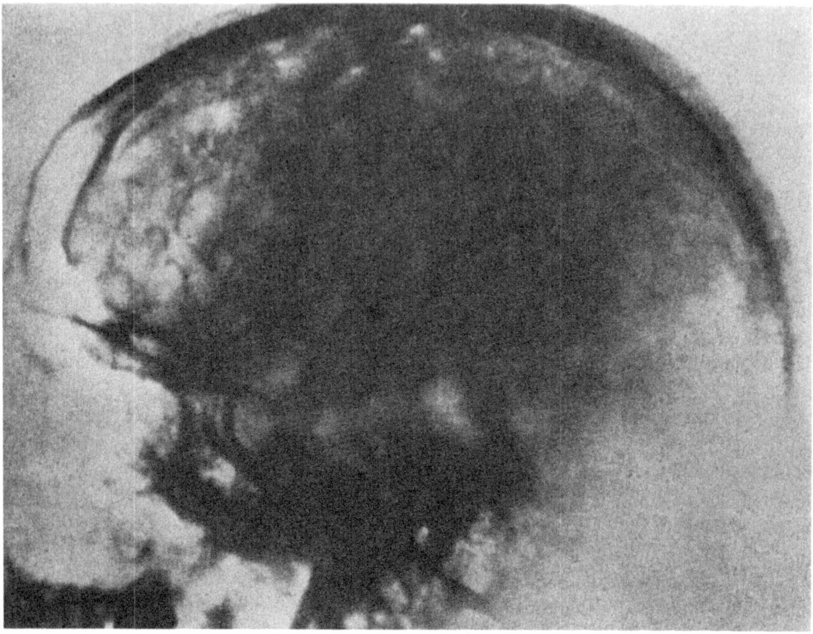

Fig 1. First Cerebral Angiogram

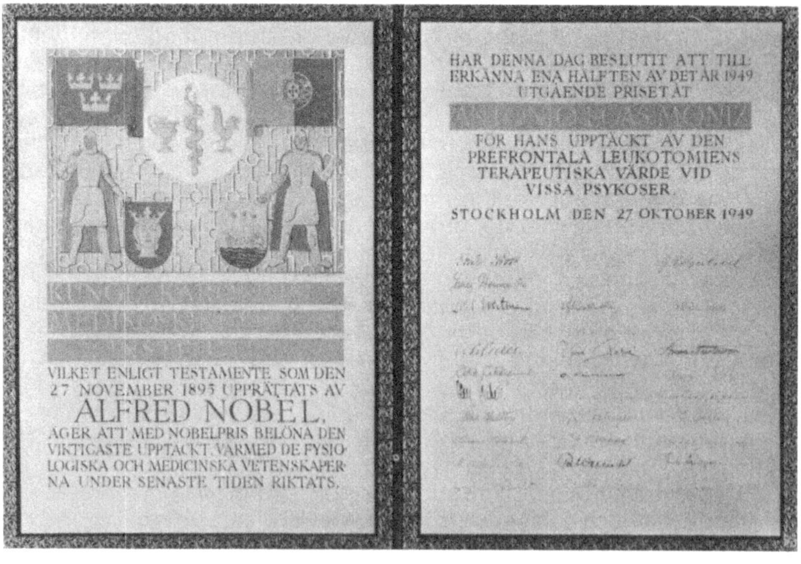

Nobel Prize Diploma

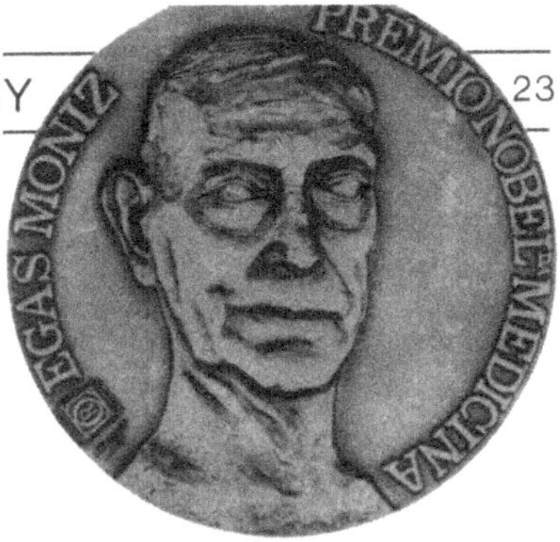

Egas Moniz
1874-1955

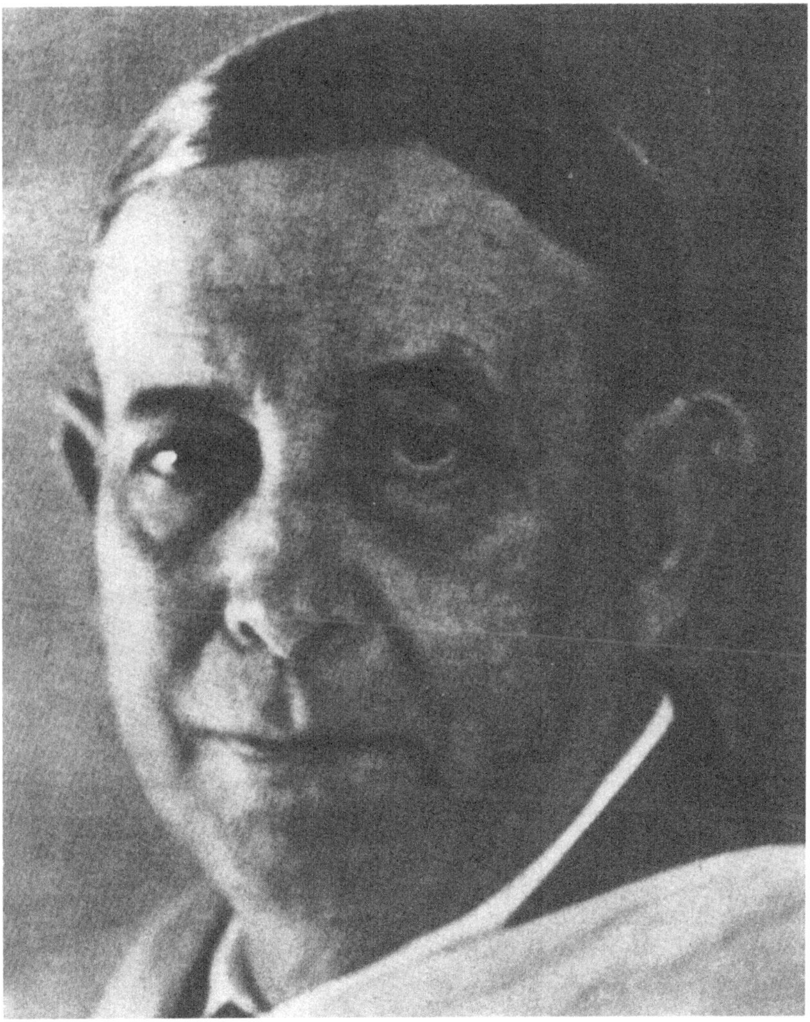

Egas Moniz
1874-1955

António Caetano de Abreu Freire Egas Moniz received in 1949 the Nobel Prize in Physiology and Medicine "for his discovery of therapeutic value of leucotomy in certain psychoses." Even if this was the manifest reason for the granting of the prize his invention of human cerebral angiography must also have been taken into account.

He was the descendant of a distinguished family and he was born in 1874, in Avanca [1] a small village in the north of Portugal.

He finished his medical studies in 1899, at the University of Coimbra, where he later became a professor of Internal Medicine. In 1911 he was transferred to Lisbon where he was appointed to the newly created Chair of Neurology. Most of his neurological training was obtained in France, first in Bordeaux with Pitres and Jean Abadie, and then in Paris where the neurological school included at the time men like Pierre Marie, Déjérine, Babinski and Brissand. Within the younger group he had a close relationship with Sicard. It is probable that his friendship with the inventor of myelography may have influenced him in the attempt to achieve diagnostic methods for lesions of the brain.

For many years (1911 to 1926) Egas Moniz divided his creative powers between neurology and politics. He made no interruption in his practice or study of neurology (in 1917 he published a large and remarkable paper on the neurology of war) and yet he was in succession Member of Parliament, Minister of Foreign Affairs, Ambassador in Madrid and President of the Portuguese Delegation to the Versailles Peace Conference.

In 1926, the establishing dictatorial government had a most fortunate consequence, that of diverting Egas Moniz from the political world. From then on he concentrated solely on the practice, study and research of neurology.

Essentially he was a clinician, and it was certainly the enormous amount of difficulty to be found in the precise diagnosis of brain tumours (demanded by Cushing's newly introduced surgical treatment) that led Egas Moniz to think about the possibility of devising the neuroradiological method on the lines of the one his friend Sicard had obtained for compressive lesions of the spinal cord.

Moniz had the intuition that inside the skull the blood vessels would be capable of X-ray opacity, thus disclosing more instructive

1) Where a museum is open to the public in a permanent exhibition of books, paintings, furniture, china, etc., that Egas Moniz collected with great taste and knowledge.

information than that available from the ventriculography developed by Dandy.

If by means of an innocuous method it could be possible to obtain an X-ray image of the several components on the intracranial vascular nets. Moniz expected not only to have a means of localizing brain tumours but also to predict their pathological nature. He also foresaw the possibility of getting anatomical and physiological data of paramount importance to the understanding of the cerebral circulation and its pathology.

With this in mind, Egas Moniz skilfully planned a number of experiments which represent a model of scientific research in that most delicate field of the human application of laboratory findings and procedures.

Several drugs expected to be harmless and radiopaque were tried. Iodides and bromides in particular were used in various concentrations. Studies in the corpse came next to determine the quality of X-ray films and to obtain the "normal" picture of cerebral arteries. Then the effect of the injections of drugs in the blood stream was carefully evaluated in dogs and monkeys. When he was convinced of the local and general safety of the drug he had chosen as contrast (sodium iodide 25%) he had the first cerebral angiography performed[2] in a patient on the 28th June 1927. Some days later (7th July) he presented to the Société Neurologique de Paris, a communication with the title: "L'encéphalographie artérielle, son importance dans la localisation des tumeurs cérébrales.

The performing of leucotomy was basically motivated, just like angiography, by the clinician's dissatisfaction with the scarcity of therapeutic agents to help his patients.

The carefully laboured decision to produce lesions in the frontal lobes to modify the behaviour of certain mental patients was certainly influenced by the detailed observation of R. Brickner (in the *Proc. Assoc. for Res. in Nerv. and Ment. Dis. 1932),* of a patient operated upon by Dandy, in whom large portions of both frontal lobes had been removed without subsequent disturbances of cognition. The work of Fulton and Jacobsen also had some part in his audacious enterprise.

2) Egas Moniz had gout since 23 years of age. This had caused great deformity of his hands and all the acts requiring manual skill were performed by one of his younger assistants.

3) This was the first publication on cerebral angiography — *Revue Neurologique* No. 1, 1927. Several others were soon to follow. The main ones are the monographies "Diagnostic des tumeurs cérébrales et épreuve de l'Encéphalographie Artérielle" Masson et Cie, Paris 1931, "L'angiographie Cérébrale" Masson et Cie., Paris 1934 and "Die cerebrale Arteriographie und Phlebographie" Julius Springer, Berlin 1940.

On the 12th November 1935, Moniz proposed to his collaborator, the neurosurgeon Almeida Lima, the performance of the destruction of portions of white matter in the frontal lobes of some mental patients by means of alcohol injections. The results were encouraging. It is not possible here to give an account of the expansion of "brain leucotomy" which is known in some countries by the unfortunate label of "psychosurgery". The several technical variations of the operation and the passionate controversies it still provokes have interfered with the development of an accepted opinion as to its indications.

Egas Moniz died suddenly on the 13th December 1955. He was 81 and had entirely retained all his mental faculties to the last moment.

Almeida Lima
Professor da Faculdade de Medicina
Lisboa, Portugal.

FIRST COMMUNICATION ON CEREBRAL ANGIOGRAPHY

Egas Moniz

(Arterial encephalography; Its importance in the location of cerebral tumours).
Revue Neurologique, No. 1, July 1927. Vol. 48 p72

To attain visualisation of the cerebral arteries, it was necessary to procure an opaque, non-oily substance which could easily pass through the capillaries in such a way as to avoid any kind of embolism, and which would be harmless. This was our primary task.

As the substance would have to be introduced via the internal carotid, however, it was necessary to know whether this artery would tolerate such introduction without disturbance and whether the brain would accept the chosen opaque substances without showing severe reactions.

Another problem to be solved was the immediate dilution of the aqueous solution by the large volume of blood, which would lead to loss of visualisation if it could not be introduced at the outset and, as far as possible, as a substitute for blood. Each systole should propel 160 cc of blood around the body and we have calculated that this amount should put between 3 and 4 cc of blood into each internal carotid. This is to say that in a period of 5 cardiac cycles, an intracarotid injection carried out during this time (4 seconds) would be dissolved in 20 cc. of blood which would make the visibility of the liquid introduced disappear.

At the same time, it was necessary to have a very good X-ray machine — which we do not have — in order to obtain pictures at a precise moment before rapid dilution takes place. In other words, temporary ligation of the carotid was essential to the procedure.

Having obtained visualisation of the arterial network, we need to have a fairly consistent normal picture. If a cerebral neoplasm is present, it should be possible to define some point or other at which it is causing displacement of fine arteries, if not any growth of the tumour, because the network should show quite appreciable changes, at least in certain regions.

In very vascular tumours it is highly probable that a visible blush could be obtained due to the penetration of liquid opaque to X-rays.

This outline which we have just presented in a general way demonstrates the path followed in our experiments.

The size of the tumours cannot be diagnosed by the severity of the general symptoms of hypertension. Every neurologist has had surprises in this connection. Large tumours, for example those of the corpus callosum[1], can grow and develop without showing appreciable disturbances.

1) Egas Moniz: (Tumours of the corpus callosum). A study which should appear in one of the forthcoming *Encéphale*.

In contrast, there are small tumours which give rise to quite remarkable hypertensive symptoms. Sometimes these develop rapidly, as if there were an inflammatory process. In other cases they appear gradually and slowly. Thus we can never relate the symptoms observed to the size of the tumour.

It would be very useful if radiographic methods of investigating the brain could give us complete information on location, growth, etc., of intracranial neoplasms. In solving this serious diagnostic problem, however, the principal objective is location of at least part of the tumour.

For example, in the tumour of the corpus callosum, to which we have referred, the callosal and calloso-marginal arteries showed changes and the left hemisphere, in which the anterior horn of the greatly dilated lateral ventricle had been invaded by the neoplasm, and the arterial circulation, also showed severe alterations.

We have considered solely the internal carotid and the arterial network derived from it, since the internal carotid gives rise to the anterior and sylvian arteries, two major arteries which irrigate the larger part of the brain, and particularly the silent part, that is to say, the region where invasion by neoplasms does not produce appreciable symptoms.

The vertebral arteries supply the diencephalon and cerebellum, where lesions are fairly easy to locate, since they are manifested by disturbances well-known to neurologists. Furthermore, they are not easily accessible and, as they irrigate the medulla oblongata, the introduction of substances can have serious and immediate consequences.

The internal carotid artery is localised to its hemisphere. The anterior communicating arteries, between the two anterior cerebral arteries and the posterior communicating arteries, branches of the basilar artery, are the only possible passages to the opposite hemisphere. Injected substances consequently remain in the circulation of the internal carotid artery concerned. The constant irrigation of the communicating arteries with blood from the internal carotid on the other side and the two vertebral arteries not only prevents the entry of the opaque substance but sends blood to the carotid which is ligated momentarily.

Of the opaque substances, we initially preferred strontium bromide, and in another article [2] we have given our conclusions on the subject.

2) Egas Moniz: Intracarotid injections and opaque substances. Presse mèdicale 1927.

Of the bromides, those of strontium and lithium are the most opaque. Sodium and potassium bromides also show good opacity. Strontium bromide is a little less toxic than lithium bromide; the latter still has advantages from this point of view as large amounts can be injected into the veins without causing disturbances. Nevertheless, lithium bromide is a little more irritant than strontium bromide and its intravenous injection in high concentration causes a painful sensation along the course of the vein, though this is transitory.

Strontium bromide, which we preferred, never caused this, but concentrated solutions, above 30 per cent, gave rise to a feeling of heat, initially localised to the head but later spreading throughout the body; it was transitory but quite disturbing. It is comparable with that produced by the intravenous injection of calcium chloride. Lithium also produces these effects but they are less severe. These feelings of heat can be avoided by giving the injections slowly.

In large doses, strontium bromide causes induration of the veins; this was corrected by the addition of 10 per cent glucose.

In this way we were able to inject solutions containing up to 80 per cent strontium bromide and in very large doses (10 to 15 cc), without disturbance to the patients.

Patients with post-encephalitic parkinsonism benefited greatly from these injections and asked for them in spite of the unpleasant sensation which they produced.

We also confirmed that 70 per cent solutions of strontium bromide were entirely harmless. With 80 per cent we observed a tendency to fainting in one male patient, which made us discontinue the use of this concentration.

We determined the opacities of the various bromides, and notably strontium bromide, from 10 to 80 per cent, by putting into a skull a carton of small rubber tubes filled with increasing concentrations of the salt. We found that the opacity from 30 per cent upwards was quite considerable, but even a 10 per cent solution was visible through the skull. We carried out experiments with this salt in animals and then in man, but we will not concern ourselves much with the results obtained.

After an accident that we had, we were led in another direction. It appeared to us that the bromides were less toxic, and in particular less irritant, than the iodides; it was because of this that we preferred them. We knew, however, that the iodides had greater opacity to X-rays than bromides, since opacity depends on atomic weight, which is much higher for iodine than for bromine . The atomic weight of the associated metal must also be taken into account, but in a general way the iodides are much more opaque than the bromides. We repeated with iodides the experiments that we had carried out with bromides and we decided on sodium iodide, which was already being used clinically by intravenous injection. When the cerebral arteries of cadavers were injected with 30 per cent, 20 per cent, 10 per cent, and even 7.5 per cent solutions, we found that they were again visible through the skull. We believe that this finding is so important that we venture to publish four arteriograms obtained with these injections. The 7.5 per cent solution demonstrates some of the larger arteries, within the limits of visibility. This finding, which was quite unexpected, could be utilised in other clinical investigations outside neurology.

We injected solutions of sodium iodide ranging from 10 to 50 per cent into the veins of humans. We found that with up to 30 per cent the injections were not painful, even when given with some speed. At 30 per cent, a few patients complained of pain along the course of the vein, and this increased and was consistently found when this concentration was exceeded. The addition of other substances (glucose, bromides, etc.) had no effect on this painful reaction. We stopped at a concentration of 25 per cent, which still gave a very good opacity and did not cause any pain on intravenous injection.

The iodides are less toxic to the tissues than the bromides. Special care must be taken in giving the injections to prevent extravasation of the solution. The iodides, however, are harmless to the arteries. Brooks, who injected them in a concentration of 100 per cent in cases of arteritis obliterans, confirmed after amputation of one of the limbs, that the arteries showed no macroscopic or microscopic lesions.

We studied other iodides but have not used them. The majority were highly unstable. Strontium and lithium iodides liberate iodine, even from low concentrations. Rubidium iodide, which is very opaque, is not toxic, but causes pain in quite low doses.

Sodium iodide is not very stable either. Above 30 per cent, liberation of iodine is almost constant, particularly if the ampoules are kept for a long time or if they are exposed to light. As a precaution we use recently-prepared solutions, if possible sterilised on the actual day of use. When the ampoules have a slightly yellowish appearance, we do not use them. The chemical purity of the salts to be used must also be borne in mind.

We carried out many experiments on animals, to determine the toxicity of the chosen compounds, to assess the effects of the substances used on the brain by giving intracarotid injections, or to capture the injected cerebral arteries in radiographs.

For determination of toxicity, we gave injections to rabbits and dogs. The results with strontium and lithium bromides and sodium iodide were completely encouraging with doses that would be used in man. Experiments carried out with intravenous and subcutaneous injections demonstrated their safety even in very high concentration.[2] We confirmed these results by giving intravenous injections to human subjects.

With intracarotid injections, we found that dogs showed great resistance to the substances introduced. We have two dogs still alive, one weighing 8 kg, which had 3 cc of a 100 per cent solution of strontium bromide injected into the carotid, and the other a bitch weighing 5.1 kg, which had an intracarotid injection of 1.5 cc of a 25 per cent solution of sodium iodide.

The carotid arteries of dogs are quite resistant to intracarotid injections, but their response varies. Sometimes haematomas form, in other cases blood spurts out after the injection, while in some animals the arteries do not show any reaction. We have never seen any troublesome complications in this connection, just as we have not observed them in man.

Dogs were the animals chosen for our radiographic studies, but they did not prove good subjects for this purpose, as the cranium shows lines on the radiogram, deriving from bony corrugations at the muscular insertions, which are very numerous and very extensive in the head of this species.

The internal carotid is very slender in the dog and we were unable to reach it directly. To do so we ligated the common carotid above its origin, at the same time pressing on the occipital artery, which in this species is as large as the internal carotid and which arises above and very close to it. However, this was not sufficient to give a radiogram of the cerebral arteries in the dog. It was necessary not to let blood pass from the common carotid, in order to avoid dilution of the opaque substance used. We therefore placed the ligature lower and injected the opaque solution into the isolated segment, which forced the solution to enter the internal carotid without mixing with blood from the common carotid.

The first radiographs were negative. They were obtained with the Potter-Bucky diaphragm and with a fairly long exposure. It was because of this that we realised that the essential condition for success was *instantaneous radiography*, to capture the passage of the substance through the arteries, now kept supplied with blood from the collaterals. The exposures which we could obtain with our hospital apparatus were still too long - a quarter of a second -but notwithstanding we succeeded in obtaining positive results. In all our experiments it was this radiological inadequacy that was the most serious problem to overcome. It was even the indirect cause of the vexations we encountered and of our not attaining positive results sooner. I hope that this situation will be improved within a short time but I do not know whether with a more powerful apparatus alone we shall attain what is essential for us. We shall return to this subject later.

In dogs, we sometimes injected 100 per cent strontium bromide and sometimes 100 per cent lithium bromide into the internal carotid and captured the pattern of some of the cerebral arteries and of the veins of the neck in three cases. These results encouraged us to continue with experiments on man.

Before going any further, we carried out studies on cadavers in order to gain an idea of the arterial tree of the brain and to define our anatomical concepts by means of our radiographs. We even took advantage of this work, which was carried out in collaboration with Almeida Dias and Almeida Lima [3], to put forward some radio-anatomical ideas and some new concepts on the topography of the skull and brain. By means of stereoscopic radiography we were able to separate the two carotid systems of the brain: the internal or anterior cerebral and the external or sylvian. (middle cerebral artery).

These experiments were most illuminating. Very good networks could be visualised by injecting, under pressure, a 100 per cent solution of sodium iodide into the internal carotid and the vertebral artery on the same side at the same time.

We obtained a large number of radiographs on cadavers in order to have a normal picture of the distribution of the arteries as seen by means of X-rays. We did everything possible to obtain the cadavers of persons who had died of brain tumours. In the form of changes in the arterial network they would have provided a partial confirmation of the

(3) Egas Moniz, Almeida Dias and Almeida Lima: Radio-arteriography and cranio-cerebral topography. Journal de Radiologie, 1927.

thesis we had put forward, but in the six months of our experiments we were not able to obtain a single cadaver which was useful for the purpose.

It was after all this work that we went on to studies in patients.

The experiments carried out underwent considerable changes as our work progressed. There was always one great difficulty to overcome: the entry of blood at the moment of the injection of the opaque solution, which led to an immediate fall in the concentration, and hence to a decrease in the possibility of obtaining visualisation of the vessels.

We had this in dogs and we overcame it by ligating the carotid artery. It must be noted, however, that in dogs the communicating vessels are not comparable with those present in man and the problem here is much more difficult to solve. But the shadows were well-defined and easy to see, and consequently to obtain a pattern of the arteries it is necessary to have: 1) a solution which is still opaque when mixed with the existing blood; 2) an X-ray machine which can make rapid enough exposures to capture the course of the liquid in the vessels.

We can divide our experiments into two stages, one concerned with injections of strontium bromide, and the other with the use of sodium iodide. We began by trying to inject into the unexposed internal carotid in man. We tried this in four cases; before that, we attempted to approach the internal carotid at the point of entry into the carotid foramen, but without success. It is possible that we did not succeed because we used very fine needles, 0.5 and 0.6mm; the blood never issued because of their small diameter and length (5 cm). We abandoned this approach and used as guides the sterno-mastoid border in the triangle formed by its border, the anterior venter of the digastric muscle, and the omo-hyoid bone.

In our *first case,* a patient with general paralysis, we had the impression that we had reached the carotid, and injected 7 cc of a 70 per cent solution of strontium bromide without effect. It is probable that the injection was given into the internal jugular vein, as the patient did not complain of pain.

In the *second case,* the injection was given into the internal carotid, and as we had the patient ready for the first radiograph to be taken, compression of the common carotid was carried out in order to prevent the entry of blood into the internal carotid during the injection of the opaque solution. There was a rather violent painful reaction after the introduction of 5 to 6 cc of the solution; the patient got up suddenly and radiography could not be carried out.

In the *third case,* a patient with parkinsonism who had benefited greatly from intravenous injections of strontium bromide, unpleasant sensations were also experienced and we decided not to continue. This patient subsequently developed a Claude Bernard-Horner syndrome, though this has since passed off completely.

The *fourth patient* gave us a rather unpleasant surprise.The needle came out of the artery and a large part of the liquid (more than 10 cc) was extravasated into the surrounding cellular tissue. There were no serious consequences; the patient had a temperature of about 38°C for a few days and absorption was slow, but there was no abscess. He developed a Claude Bernard-Horner syndrome, but this improved gradually. After this accident, we decided surgical exposure of the artery should be used. Surgeon M. Antonio Martins was kind enough to undertake to expose and inject into the internal carotid.

The *fifth case* was a female patient aged 20 years with a cerebral neoplasm which had not been localised. She was blind. When the internal carotid had been exposed, it was ligated and a 70 per cent solution of strontium bromide was injected. The artery was punctured twice and about 4 cc of liquid was injected. From the outset the patient complained. She had a background of neuropathy and became very agitated. Later she developed a type of anaesthesia with speech disturbances and, after a minute's interval, she ceased to speak. There were no other adverse effects. The radiographs were negative; they were taken too late. The injections had no unpleasant sequelae for the patient; she had fever (39°C) on the following day and transitory dysphagia, but by the third day she was well again.

The patient in the *sixth case* was aged 48 and had very severe post-encephalitic parkinsonism. He had great muscular rigidity, tremors, transitory diplopia, retropulsion with repeated falls blepharospasm, and great difficulty in speaking. Scopolamine had not benefited him. Intravenous injections of high concentrations of strontium bromide had brought about improvement. We selected him with the two-fold aim of obtaining arterial radiograms and of seeing the result of the direct action of strontium bromide on the brain. When the carotid artery had been exposed and ligated, 13 to 14 cc of a strontium bromide solution was injected. The patient complained of severe pain. With the object of obtaining four radiograms, we kept the ligature in place for 2 minutes. The first radiograph, which was shaky, nonetheless showed that the opaque fluid had entered the artery. A further radiogram, taken immediately afterwards, showed only the injected internal carotid and a small opacity in the upper part of the anterior cerebral artery, which demonstrated that a thrombus had formed immediately in this artery. Another radiogram, taken at the time the ligature was removed from the carotid, visualised the sylvian and, in particular, the posterior cerebral artery, which demonstrated to us that the pressure of the carotid blood had crossed the stream coming from the vertebral artery. As the blood could not have passed via the anterior cerebral artery, the pressure had been, on the one hand, on the field of the vertebral artery and, on the other hand, on the ophthalmic artery. The patient subsequently developed a thrombophlebitic syndrome and died 8 hours after the injection. The state of this patient's arteries would have played a part in the occurrence of this accident [4], but we committed an error of technique in maintaining the ligation of the internal carotid too long and after the injection. The large dose of the substance must also have been a disadvantage, but we cannot explain the immediate formation of the thrombus in the anterior cerebral artery, which we have never observed in animals. Can the vascular and perivascular lesions in severe encephalitis explain its formation under the influence of the bromide?

This accident made us abandon bromide solutions and consider the iodides, with the aim of obtaining adequate opacification with lower doses than those used with the bromides.

It was at this time that we commenced a study of the opacity of the iodides and their action on tissues and vessels. As we have already stated, sodium iodide solutions are visible through the skull even in very low concentrations, such as, for example, 10 per cent or even 7.5 per cent, and sodium iodide solutions up to 50 per cent can be injected intravenously without adverse effect. The injections are not painful with solutions up to 30 per cent.

In the circumstances we chose 22 to 25 per cent solutions for intra-carotid injections. The dose which could be injected without danger to the patient and which would give the required opacification had to be determined. For this we were convinced that large volumes of liquid were not necessary, because when it entered the circulation of the communicating arteries (the internal carotid being ligated), the larger part of the substance would disappear. The amount to be introduced should be such that, when mixed with the blood contained

4) Histopathological examination of the brain, under the supervision of Professor Pereira, has not yet been completed.

in the part of the carotid above the ligature, it would give a solution of about 20 per cent, which would still be opaque. For this, it would be necessary to inject 3 to 5 cc of a 25 per cent solution of sodium iodide and towards the end make the radiographic exposure while the injection is continued.

As the X-ray machine in use at our hospital only gives exposures of ¼ second, we went as far as to give 5 cc of the solution.

This solution, probably 20 per cent in concentration, comes into contact with blood which comes either from the anterior communicating artery or from the posterior communicating artery. We cannot know the volume of blood which these arteries return to the circulation of the hemisphere as a substitute for the blood from the internal carotid. We have calculated however, that for each cardiac cycle, they would provide at the most the volume of blood corresponding to the volume of solution injected in a second, that is to say, about 1 cc. But under these conditions, solution would not occur immediately, the two liquids, blood and iodide solution, going along side by side. An opacity of 10 per cent would be obtained, which would be sufficient to visualise some, at least, of the larger arteries of the brain. It would only be necessary to capture the progress of the liquid by making very rapid exposures.

We tried intracarotid injections of 22 per cent sodium iodide (first case) and of 25 per cent solutions, without any adverse effects on the patients. We carried this out in 4 cases, but one of these does not count, because a poor artery was injected and the experiment was abandoned without radiography being performed. In the other three cases the injections were given into the internal carotid without adverse effects, sodium iodide being used in the concentrations indicated.

The *first case,* a patient suffering from a cerebral neoplasm suspected of being localised to the right fronto-parietal region because of a slight opacity detected by radiography, blind in the right eye and seeing very little with the left eye, was injected with 3 cc of a 22 per cent solution of sodium iodide. He underwent local anaesthesia with Novocain and beforehand an injection of morphine hydrochloride with 0.5 mg of atropine sulphate was given. At the moment of obtaining the radiograph the ligature was removed from the carotid with the intention of profiting from the entry into the cerebral circulation of the opaque mass which was accumulating in the carotid pool. The result would have been positive if we had had available the means of making very rapid exposures, but with ¼ second and with the speed of blood coming from the carotid, the image disappeared without leaving any radiographic trace.

In the sixth case of the bromide series, with this procedure we obtained the pattern of the sylvian and posterior cerebral arteries. Visualisation of the posterior cerebral artery was found to be the greater, probably because the opposition of the stream of blood coming from the basilar artery held back for a moment the stream coming from the internal carotid, making it appreciably visible.

Radiography in the first case in the iodide series was completely negative, there being no sign of visualisation of the arteries.

When the internal carotid was injected, the patient's pulse-rate fell from 90 to 56, but his only complaint was of slight pain in the ear. On the following day he showed some dysphagia and his temperature rose to 38°C. On the third day he got up and since then he has remained unwell.

The *second patient,* a blind man who had been under our care for several years with cranial hypertension, showed no obvious signs of localisation. There were no cerebellar symptoms, but he had very marked nystagmus, even when the eyes were in the mid-position. The patient had generalised epileptic fits, affecting more the left side, which made us decide to carry out the sodium iodide test on the right. Recently he had put on some weight, but there were no other symptoms. With this information, it seemed impossible to localise the lesion. Local anaesthesia was obtained with Novocain and the carotid artery was exposed and injected before being ligated. Entry of blood into the syringe was very violent, and into 5 cc of a 25 per cent solution (of sodium iodide) were drawn in 3 cc of blood, which made the concentration fall to about 15 per cent. This is to say that if 1 cc of the solution entered the communicating arteries, and even if radiography were carried out between two cardiac cycles, a hypothesis which has not been put forward, the concentration would be reduced to 7.5 per cent, which is the limit for visualisation in the cadaver.

However, in the radiograph the internal carotid could be seen quite well up to the upper curve. It did not appear to be normal and we even had a suspicion that it was of this shape because of pressure from a neoplasm, but as the other arteries could not be seen, there was no guarantee of this.

The passage of blood from the communicating arteries carried away the contents. The wave of blood probably passed at the moment radiography was being carried out, and the shadow given by the sodium iodide, which was already much delayed, was lost during the time needed to obtain the picture.

During the injection this patient complained of transitory pain in the temples, which was not very severe, and also slight pain in the right eye and ear. There was a fall in pulse-rate from 95 to 60 during the injection. Slight dysphagia on the following day. On the third day he got up and could eat without difficulty.

The *third patient* in the iodide series was a man of 20 with a pituitary tumour. He was a typical case of the Fröhlich-Babinski syndrome. He was blind and latterly had had severe attacks of vomiting and headache. His condition was grave.

In this patient a good technique was used for the first time: the internal carotid was exposed and the injection was given before ligation, because after this was done it was very difficult to achieve. Blood was not allowed to enter the syringe [5] and ligation was rapidly carried out. Five cc of a 25 per cent solution of sodium iodide was injected and the ligature immediately removed. The patient had no ill effects. There was no fall in pulse rate. There was slight dysphagia on the following day. After the third day he was well.

This patient had been given two injections of 10 mg of morphine and atropine during the three quarters of an hour before the injection of sodium iodide.

The radiogram (Fig. 1) shows the carotid artery pulled forward and without the upper curve. The sylvian artery, which is well visible, is also drawn forwards and upwards. The anterior cerebral artery shows a different arrangement from that seen in normal network and is very slender and somewhat obliterated.

The tumour is the cause of the changes in position of the internal carotid and of the sylvian artery and probably of the changes in the anterior cerebral artery, but on this point we cannot give a definite opinion. This will all be displayed when these radiographs are compared with normal ones.

Our thesis has thus been proved. It is possible to obtain radio-arteriograms of the brain in living people and they can provide aids to the localisation of tumours. It is only necessary to carry out experiments to obtain information which a single case cannot provide.

The technique is simple, but it is possible that many modifications will be introduced. It will even be possible to make the

5) A stop-cock device with two syringes can be used, one filled with physiological saline and connected to the needle at the time the artery is punctured and the other filled with the substance to be injected. We used this in the first few injections, which were carried out on the unexposed artery.

injection with the artery unexposed, using compression of the common carotid, either digitally or by means of a compressor of the type described by Dupuytren. This will depend on the concentration of the solution to be introduced. Analgesia with morphine should be substituted for anaesthesia with ethylchloride or nitrous oxide if high concentrations are used.

The meningeal arteries, coming from the external carotid, could also be examined by injecting that artery. By giving the injection into the common carotid both networks might be obtained (meningeal and cerebral), and these are very easy to distinguish in the radio-arteriograms.

The great problem to be solved, however, is not now that of intracarotid injection and the concentrations to be used, as these have more or less been determined. The radiological technique is much more important. It could give rise to much simplification and to new concepts of vascular encephalography, because not only the arterial network could be visualised, but also the veins and sinuses.

Several exposures must be obtained very rapidly, as it is known that the blood flow is at a rate of 10 metres per second, and it is essential for them to be in succession. It would be very interesting and very practical - because pictures would never be lost - to make an actual cinematograph film of the cerebral circulation with these opaque substances in motion. There is also another problem to be solved: stereoscopic radiograms which are obtained very rapidly so as not to lose the movement of the opaque solutions in the arteries. Solving this problem seems a little more difficult to us, but to obtain a good picture of the displacement of arteries by the pressure of tumours, stereoscopy would be a valuable aid.

This is to say that at the moment the problem goes over to radiology, which - we believe - will fulfil all our hopes within a short time. We will be continuing our experiments, but we need a better X-ray machine. Without that, progess will not be appreciable.

At the moment, the technique we recommend as being harmless to the patients and capable of giving a fairly good arterial encephalogram, is as follows:-

1) Prepare the patient by giving one or two injections of morphine and atrophine;
2) Expose the internal carotid artery;
3) Fix the patient's head to the photographic frame by means of a bandage,to avoid movements of the head;
4) Puncture the carotid artery without letting blood enter the syringe;
5) Always take great care to prevent air from entering;
6) Immediately use forceps to act as a temporary ligature of the internal carotid artery;
7) Immediately and rapidly inject 5 to 6 cc of a 25 per cent solution of sodium iodide, recently prepared and sterilised;
8) Make one or more radiographic exposures (as rapidly as possible) while continuing to inject the opaque solution.
9) Immediately remove the temporary ligature from the internal carotid artery.

Acknowledgements

We have already mentioned some of our collaborators in our articles. We must also thank our friends Assistant Eduardo Coelho, who always attended on us in our clinical trials, Professor Cancela d'Abreu, Assistants R. Loff and L. Pacheco, and Drs. A. Fernandes and M. Beirao for the assistance they gave during the course of this work.

THE FIRST COMMUNICATION ON AORTOGRAPHY AND ARTERIOGRAPHY OF THE LIMBS

Reynaldo dos Santos

Arteriography of the limbs, with the assistance of Augusto Lamas and J. Pereira Caldas.
A Medicina Contemporanea, 1929

The introduction of arteriography as a new technique took place in 1927 thanks to the work of Prof. Egas Moniz who succeeded in his attempts to visualise the cerebral circulation and to use this achievement in the diagnosis of cerebral tumours. Sicard himself recognised that the technique marked a new era in the diagnosis of vascular disorders of the brain.

It is for the neurologists to define the scope of this technique. Although highly specialised, cerebral arteriography is only one aspect of the visualisation of arteries and we are proud of the fact that Portuguese science, which is unfortunately so short of original ideas, is in the lead in one of the most delicate areas of visualisation of arteries, which requires precise technique derived from the experimental research which justifies its use in clinical practice.

It was this technique which we used for the first arteriographies which we carried out and we are well aware that we owe the success of our first attempts to the technique which Professor Egas Moniz defined and which essentially we still use today.

For all practical purposes Egas Moniz pioneered the technique which we use. We use sodium iodide as the contrast medium because it gives a good shadow in arteriography of the limbs as it does in cerebral arteriography. Our results for pyeloscopy and pyelography are also due to the choice of this medium since it is one of the most radio-opaque and least irritant of the fluids usually employed. We never use the quickly absorbed contrast medium for visualising arteries that Sicard does; we do not think it is a good thing to use it because not only does it give irregular shadows but also it may cause gangrene by blocking the capillaries.[1] A concentration of 25% sodium iodide is, with a few exceptions, the best, for its opacity is good and it is not very painful. The 100% concentration used by Brooks is so painful that general anaesthesia is required.

In our patients we use only local anaesthesia for finding the artery.

Large amounts of the 25% sodium iodide solutions can be used without trouble; we have on occasion injected 40 cc without the least evidence of iodism or intolerance. These doses were given intravenously for therapeutic purposes with no trouble.

In our opinion the dose can be even higher since after being introduced into an artery the fluid is fixed in the tissues served by the artery and is only absorbed later, returning little by little into the circulation. We have performed serial arteriographies which confirm this. Using the same radiographic technique, timing, intensity and

1) Harvier and Lemaire, *Bul. Soc. Med. Hopitaux.* Paris, 1927.

current it is possible to discern in the X-ray negatives (but not in positive prints because in these the quality is degraded) that at the same time as the opaque fluid is disappearing in the arteries an opacity appears in the tissues, like a slight loss of transparency and this corresponds with fixation of the sodium iodide.

There were no local disorders in the patients we injected except for slight and transient pain felt by the patients during the injection. In fact the patients' pain from their diseases became less severe when the iodide was given; others have also noticed this. One of our patients had a very painful arthritis of his wrist which prevented any movement; after the injection the pain stopped and he was able to move the joint with very little pain.

The amount of the solution to be used depends on the extent of the area to be visualised.

An injection of 10 cc may be enough for the upper limb or lower leg but it is not enough for a thigh or the whole lower limb and the amount should be increased to 20 cc or even 30 cc.

Arterial puncture presents very little trouble. When the needle is removed a few drops of blood usually come out of the hole but a simple dressing is enough for all to return to normal. In one case only, a small but persistent spurt of blood was stopped with an adrenaline solution. The X-rays should be taken *during the course of the injection,* when the fluid has nearly all been injected. The solution should be introduced into the artery as fast as possible and for this reason wide-bore needles should be used. By this means it is possible to prevent the fluid being diluted too much by the flow of blood. In an attempt to retain the solution in the arteries for longer and to achieve improved arteriographs we tried to delay the circulation by compressing the roots of the limbs (proximal to the injection) with elastic; by taking serial X-rays we were able to follow the disappearance of the arterial shadows. We found that the solution stayed in the vessels much longer but the difference in visualisation was small after 3 minutes and there was no difference after 17 minutes. In an attempt to find some alternative to compression with elastic which made it impossible to inject into the root of a limb we ligated the artery and vein temporarily just before taking the X-rays. We tried the experiment in one patient of ligating the external iliac artery and injecting into the femoral artery in Scarpa's triangle against the direction of the flow of blood in an attempt to see whether the artery was permeable at the level of ligature. We were unable to see the part in question because the iodide escaped into the collateral

vessels between the injection site and the ligature of the artery.
We carried out 10 arteriographs in 5 patients, 2 under general anaesthesia and 3 under local.

The point of this first publication at the present juncture in our investigations is to demonstrate the first possibilities of visualising the arterial circulation in the limbs and to give some insight into what a useful tool this technique will certainly be in surgical diagnosis in the future. The progress of radiological techniques in diagnosis is ever more impressive. There are now very few organs which cannot be examined either directly by their relative opacities (lung, heart, liver etc.) or by the use of opaque substances (digestive tract, urinary tract, kidneys etc.).

Others can be shown up indirectly by making use of their excretory functions such as the kidney or gall-bladder. Yet others can be examined indirectly by rendering their arterial system momentarily opaque as is the case now with the brain and as will certainly be the case with other organs which have so far evaded systematic radiological investigation.

Visualising arteries is more exciting than most authors have realised. It is of direct importance to the study of the vascular system i.e. to lesions therein (aneurysms, ruptures, obstructions, etc.) and to disorders of its function spasm, inadequate supply, development of collaterals, etc.) and it is of perhaps even greater indirect importance in the investigation of the visceral lesions which it demonstrates, as foreseen by Egas Moniz, in the diagnosis of cerebral tumours. It is this new sphere of arterial visualisation which has perhaps the greatest future and it is not the least of its merits that it deserves to carry the name of the Portuguese who conceived and executed it.

We should now compare arteriography of the limbs (by Sicard and Brooks) against the visceral arteriography of Egas Moniz for which we are trying to develop new applications among the abdominal organs.

In the light of the experience we have of paravertebral sympathetic anaesthesia and knowing how easy it is to approach the aorta and vena cava and being also aware that although accidental puncture of these vessels is frequent, it is rarely followed by serious consequences, we can foresee deliberate aortic puncture for the injection of sodium iodide followed immediately by radiography. We can then visualise at least part of the abdominal circulation (coeliac axis, renal and mesenteric arteries) and thereby obtain some idea of the nature and site of any lesions, particularly tumours (of the kidney, pancreas, liver, stomach, etc.) when the morbid anatomy of such lesions has caused definite changes in the anatomy of the vessels.

Although our preliminary attempts have so far proven quite harmless, we cannot claim to have achieved the desired objective. We wish to emphasise however, that 1) aortic puncture is quite possible and perfectly safe if the technique is based on the method used for sympathetic anaesthesia as modified in the manner suggested by studies on cadavers carried out by one of our Registrars F. Levy; 2) the injection of iodide is tolerated perfectly well; 3) the injected material has been seen by radiography to diffuse so quickly in the arteries of the abdomen and to cause such a fleeting opacity that it cannot be caught on radiographs.

We have been able to carry out one of the techniques which are necessary for the achievement of our ambition; aortic puncture and iodide injection do have therapeutic implications just like those which we have established for the limbs and which will be the subject of a later article. Further studies are required and these are being undertaken.

The technique started in Portugal is on its way and we believe that visceral arteriography is of even greater diagnostic significance than arteriography of the limbs because the scope for the diagnosis of disorders of the cranial, thoracic and abdominal organs is so great when the changes in the vessels brought about by the lesions can be visualised.

In general, visualisation has been used in arterial obstruction by the common gangrenes, in Buerger's disease, etc. for assessing the degree of obstruction and whether any collateral circulation is present. In this context it is compared to oscillometry.

Singleton has recently used the technique in arterial and arterio-venous aneurysms (one of them in the humerus). The results in gangrene have been poor and there was indeed one death from moist gangrene. We are of the opinion that visualisation of arteries has a great future in all these disorders of anatomy or function of the circulation of the limbs:

1. Arteritis and arterial obstruction. Embolism, gangrene.
2. All types of aneurysm (investigation of cause and collateral circulation).
3. Ligations of vessels (collateral circulation).
4. Sutures of vessels (it is the only way to be certain about permeability).
5. Volkmann's paralysis.
6. Arterial spasm.
7. To follow the results of sympathectomy.
8. In tumours of the limbs.
9. In inflammatory lesions.

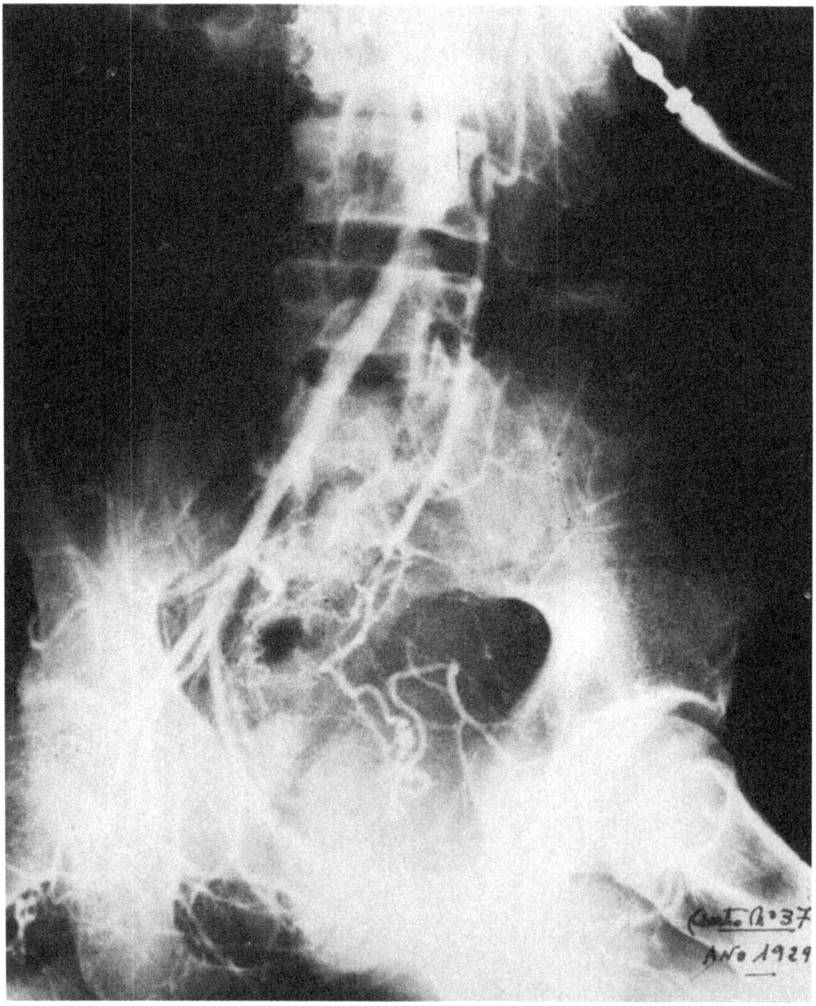

First demonstration of occlusion of the iliac arteries. Gangrene of a left toe. Obliteration of the left iliac arteries and common femoral artery. Obliteration of the inferior mesenteric artery.
Dos Santos Collection No. 37. By kind permission of the Royal College of Surgeons of Edinburgh.

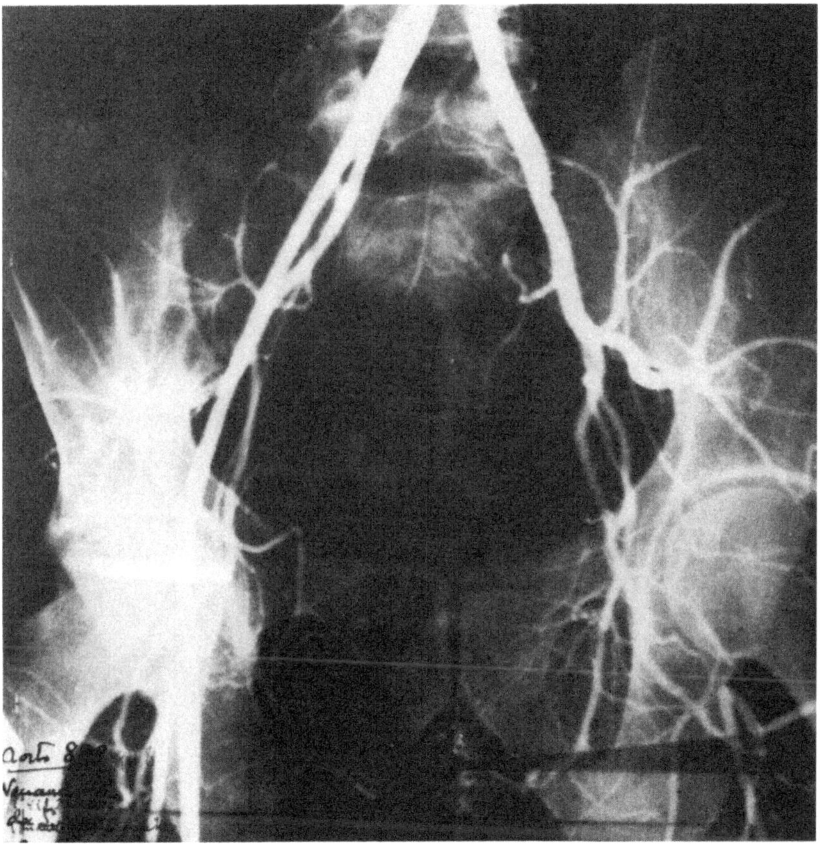

Obliteration of the external iliac and superficial femoral arteries. After an attempt of a simultaneous arteriography of both lower limbs with puncture of both common femorals, this one is the first attempt to obtain a complete aorto-arteriogram. An X-ray set, and a portable tube were used for the abdomen and the limbs, separated by a lead screen hanging from the ceiling. A complete aorto-arteriogram was obtained later with three X-ray sets.
Dos Santos Collection No. 828. By kind permission of the Royal College of Surgeons, Edinburgh.

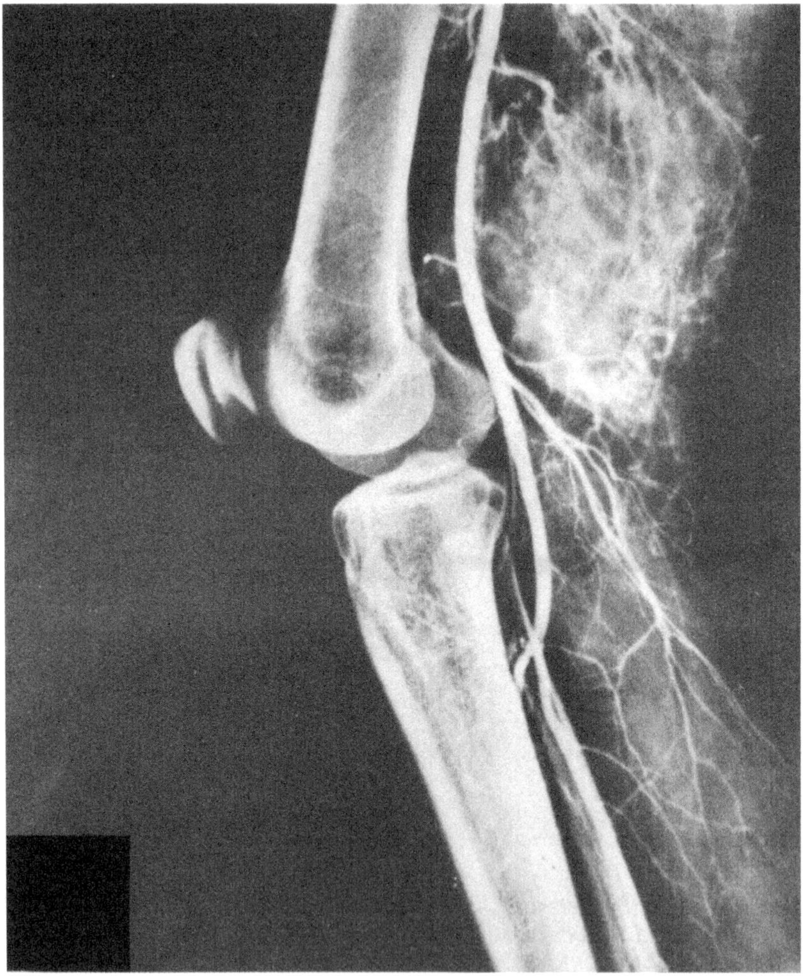

Sarcoma of the soft parts of the left thigh. One of the most beautiful early examples of the "anarchic" arterial circulation of sarcomas and of the early and elective venous return.
Dos Santos Collection No. 329. By kind permission of the Royal College of Surgeons.

SECOND COMMUNICATION ON ARTERIOGRAPHY OF THE AORTA AND THE ABDOMINAL VESSELS

Reynaldo dos Santos
Professor, Faculty of Medicine, Lisbon, Surgeon to the Hospitals.

Augusto Lamas, Surgeon to the Hospitals.
J. Pereira Caldas, Radiologist at Arroios Hospital

An excerpt from a communication at the Society for Medical Sciences, Lisbon at a meeting on 9th March, 1929.

In our first recently published article "The arteriography of the limbs" (Med. Contemp.) of January 1929 we were determined to put forward the view, which has guided our investigations, that arteriography is not merely a way of checking on the patency of vessels (nearly the only use to which it has been put so far); we wanted to get over the broader concept that it is a general diagnostic technique which is used to see and examine abnormalities by visualising their blood supply. Taking this broader view, we wanted arteriography to be extended to include the abdominal organs and in that first article we referred to our first attempts at visualising the aorta and its branches to the organs.

We can confirm and demonstrate today that this objective has been achieved and we intend to publish the first results of abdominal arteriography.

The major problem was puncturing the aorta.

Aortic puncture is now practicable and is as safe and harmless as lumbar puncture.

What were the grounds which justified our attempts?

Leaving to one side the attempts during experimental surgery which were carried out for a variety of reasons and even the results of puncturing other arteries without mishap, we will consider mainly the experience gained from anaesthesia of the splanchnic nerves, whether performed through the back or through the abdomen (Braun, Finsterer).

The aorta and the vena cava can now be reached in error and this has not been followed by mishaps either.

Examination of the region immediately after the puncture by various surgeons (Finsterer and a discussion about Heitz-Boyer's communication at the Urology Congress at Out, 1928) showed that these accidental punctures were safe. We ourselves deliberately punctured the aorta in order to give an intra-arterial injection of methylene blue as a supplement to laparotomy for tuberculous peritonitis. Fifteen days later at the post mortem (the patient died of pulmonary tuberculosis) there was no trace of a haematoma or any lesion attributable to the puncture. This shows the importance of the aorta's tunica media which rapidly closed the hole.

We therefore thought that the technique for splanchnic anaesthesia during which the vessels are punctured accidentally, could be used to enter them deliberately. With some small changes to the technique we could safely enter the aorta to the left of the mid-line.

Site of puncture. This can be at various levels depending on which vessels are to be X-rayed.

1. Above the coeliac axis, at the level of the 12th thoracic vertebra. This is essential for injecting the coeliac axis and superior mesenteric artery.

2. Above the renal arteries, at the level of the 1st lumbar vertebra.

3. Above the inferior mesenteric at the level of the 2nd lumbar vertebra.

4. Finally, above the origin of the common iliac arteries at the bifurcation of the aorta which the aortograms show should be carried out near the lower end of the body of L.3. Puncturing the aorta at this level is adequate for showing the bifurcation. This may be satisfactory for showing the iliac vessels but when the circulation in the pelvis is being examined with a view to making a diagnosis it is desirable to show the inferior mesenteric also since its branches so often are important in relation to lesions of the pelvic organs.

The levels at which aortic puncture and injection are most commonly carried out are at the bodies of T.12, L.1 and L.2 in order to visualize the coeliac axis, the renal arteries and the inferior mesenteric and iliac arteries respectively.

All these sites can be reached through the same puncture site in the skin. This site is below the 12th rib and about 8 cm. from the mid-line or one finger away from the lumbo-sacral mass. The needle is pointed toward the appropriate vertebral body; this usually means towards the spine to reach L.2, slanted more upwards for L.1 and parallel to the 12th rib and close to it for T.12.

The vertebral body is an essential reference point; after this has been found, the needle is withdrawn a little so that it can take a more anterior direction; it is then inserted further until at about 12 cm. it reaches the aorta.

The course of the descending aorta is to the left of the mid-line and obliquely downwards and inwards; it is more readily accessible in the lower part of the thorax. The higher it goes, the larger is its diameter, the further from the mid-line its position and the narrower the vertebral bodies overlying it. These factors combine to make lower thoracic puncture easier.

The only drawback to this is that the posterior margin of the lung may be in the way but this has been passed through without mishap.

We have attempted injection of the thoracic aorta at the level of T.10 because it is an easier and more reliable way of showing the uppermost branches of the abdominal aorta, particularly the coeliac axis. At this level the skin should be punctured nearer the mid-line, 3 fingers from the spinous process of T.10.

The needle should first be pointed at the vertebral body and, when this has been found, toward the para-vertebral region.

The indication that the aorta has been reached, apart from the distance (which is about 12 cm.), is the rapid flow of bright red blood which is quite different from venepuncture. This is the time to alter the syringe and to inject the opaque solution under great pressure.

The radio-opaque solution is always pure sodium iodide made up to 100% solution in water.

The needles are 12 to 14 cm. long and 1.2 mm. in diameter. Narrower needles bend easily and the sense of direction is lost. Furthermore the lumen is not large enough to allow a sufficiently large enough amount of radio-opaque material to be injected into the blood-stream for radiography to be satisfactory.

One essential point about the technique, which is the secret of success when carrying out arteriography in a flowing circulation, is that the X-rays should be of short exposure (8/10 of a second) when the blood is at its most opaque. This is brought about partly by the concentration of the solution but also by the speed of the injection i.e. the concentration of iodide in blood per unit time.

Since the arterial circulation is so rapid, the vessels are only opaque for a very short time and the solution is taken almost instantly to vessels a long way from the injected vessel. This is why what happens just before the X-rays are taken is so important. Maximum clarity can be achieved with minimum doses if the X-rays are taken almost as the injection is started. The injection should be given as fast as possible and so the syringe must be very well calibrated, ready to give the injection and well greased. It is better still to use a form of pump, as we do, which allows us to regulate the speed. We apply elastic tourniquets to the tops of the thighs in the hope of restricting the circulation of the solution to the abdominal vessels.

The injection of a 100% solution is painful and anaesthesia is required not only so that the patients can tolerate the procedure but also so that they will keep still which is necessary when the X-rays are taken. We prefer spinal root anaesthesia because not only does this facilitate puncture and injection but also it is better than general anaesthesia at ensuring immobility of the abdomen and the halting of respiration effects.

Apart from those due to spinal root anaesthesia, we have not seen any deleterious effects from puncture of the aorta or injection of the solution which we have had the opportunity of performing more than once in the same patient. Extravasation of iodide outside the aorta has been demonstrated by radiography and is mainly caused by inexperience during the first few attempts or by the patient moving; so far there have been no significant consequences. Persistent pain requires the administration of an opiate. These extravasations are always tolerated much better than those of neo-salvarsan outside a vein. In our early attempts when we took the X-rays after the injection of a particular amount of iodide solution, we used to give very large doses, 30 or 35 grams. Now we time the injection and the radiography to take place almost simultaneously and the doses are much lower. We have obtained fine arteriograms with only 10 c.c. of the solution.

The body's tolerance of high doses injected into the aorta is remarkable and has implications for treatment. The fact that higher doses are tolerated when these are given into an artery rather than into a vein was investigated and confirmed a long time ago. There are, for example, the investigations into cocaine carried out by Maxwell (1902 and 1905) which were confirmed by Weigand and those of Oppel (1909) confirmed by Goyannes (Acad. Med. Cir. Espanola, 2nd December 1912). Oppel states that a dose of cocaine is 8 to 10 times less toxic when injected into the vena cava. In arteries toxicity is inversely proportional to the size of the capillary network supplied by the artery. Thus, provided there is no stasis, the same dose will be less toxic in the aorta than in the radial artery. This is an interesting and only apparently paradoxical fact.

Radiological technique. The voltage and current depend on the region to be X-rayed.

We always use the Potter-Bucky apparatus which gives clearer films without any problems with the short time of exposure.

We have tried having the patients lying down on their backs and on their stomachs. The position of the patient depends on whether the region to be X-rayed is anterior or posterior. A vessel which is a long way from the film will give a diffuse or almost imperceptible shadow. The kidneys and even the aorta itself are best seen with the patient lying on his back. A comparison of X-rays taken in the 2 positions clearly shows that films must be interpreted in the light of the patient's position.

We will not make this article any longer by identifying all the branches of this very extensive vascular network. Suffice it to point out the blood supply to the pelvis, particularly the hypogastric and to follow the distal branches such as the gluteal, sciatic, obturador and the internal pudendal as far as the dorsal arteries of the penis and corpora cavernosa. Clearly a three-dimensional view, which we are going to obtain, will help even more with the interpretation and identification of the vessels.

In this preliminary article we wish to make it clear that radiography of the aorta and its branches in the living patient is now definitely and beyond any doubt available for the investigation of abdominal disorders. It is now possible to examine the various presentations to which the numerous disorders of the abdomen give rise. Considering only the kidney, it is easy to foresee that radiography will make it simple to diagnose tumours and horse-shoe kidney and to define the role of abnormal vessels in hydronephrosis etc. In a more general way, new avenues are open for investigating the differential diagnosis of tumours in the abdomen because its vasular connections are the best means of identifying the site and origin of a tumour.

These are the first attempts and the consistency with which the aorta can be reached and visualised is remarkable. The technique is in its early stages but we are trying to perfect it. We are able to regulate the speed of the injection with greater precision than can be achieved with a syringe and manual pressure. The constant pressure apparatus allows the speed, i.e. the dilution of the radio-opaque material by blood, to be regulated. We are trying to reduce the concentration of the solution so that is is less painful and tolerable without anaesthesia because local anaesthesia is adequate for aortic puncture.

Finally, one of us is in the process of arranging stereoscopic radiography which will be a great help in the identification of the vessels and their anatomical relationships. In our next article we will discuss the implications and therapeutic applications of arteriography using the route previously described by Goyannes. For the moment we wish to emphasize that arteriography of the aorta and its abdominal branches is not merely a method of investigating symptoms in the abdomen i.e. of examining the vascular system and the changes caused in it which can demonstrate, localise and identify disease. Arteriography throws light on the topographical anatomy of the circulation within the abdomen which can be reviewed in the light of the results of a technique which reveals the normal relationships in the living person in the absence of the changes brought about by dissection and death; in the abdomen the anatomy is very different in the living and in the dead. However, we have a new insight into the pathological anatomy of the circulation in inflammatory disorders and particularly in tumours which is not devoid of implications for diagnosis. When the problem of cinematographic radiology has been overcome the physiology of the circulation itself can be filmed, because of the transient opacity of the blood, and then it can be examined in detail in slow motion.

DISCUSSION ON AORTOGRAPHY

Reynaldo dos Santos A. Lamas J. Pereira Caldas

Arteriography of the abdominal aorta and visualisation of the relevant organs.
An excerpt from a communication at the Society for Medical Sciences, Lisbon
at a meeting on 9th March, 1929.

On his own behalf and in the names of his colleagues Mr. A. Lamas and Mr. J. Pereira Caldas, Professor Reynaldo dos Santos showed a series of arterial radiographs which had been achieved by the injection of sodium iodide. He showed examples of arteriographs of the limbs not only from cases of arterial obstruction and gangrene, but also from cases of tuberculosis of the bone, syphilis, tumours, Volkmann's disorder etc.

He broadened the scope of the technique of visualising arteries by radiography by extending it to the abdomen and showing the aorta which had not previously been done.

The appearance of the abdominal organs on X-rays is a new factor and now the fine details of their blood supply can be investigated.

By the use of this technique a diagnosis had been made in a case of renal tuberculosis in which the diagnosis had previously been in doubt.

Radiography of the arteries was attempted in 1923 by Sicard in France and later in 1924 by Brooks in America but it had only been used in the investigation of gangrene.

Professor Egas Moniz extended the use of arteriography to cerebral tumours and, by mastering the technique, he was responsible for the development of cerebral arteriography.

A much broader field is now open to the technique because in addition to arterial obstructions and most diseases of the bones and joints and tumours, it is now possible with injection of the aorta, to visualise most abdominal disorders. He mentioned finally that this technique can be used for the treatment of these disorders. He gave examples of cases of osteomyelitis, articular tuberculosis and meningo-encephalitis which had been markedly improved and even cured, which gives greater scope for treatment using the arterial route.

Mr. Egas Moniz warmly applauded the work presented by his colleagues which affords new possibilities for diagnosis and treatment. He (Moniz) was pursuing similar investigations, but remaining in the neurological field where there was still much work to be done. He congratulated those other Portuguese doctors who, with great discernment, were applying arteriography to diagnosis in other regions of the body. The results achieved by Reynaldo dos Santos, Lamas and José Caldas were quite remarkable.

Injection of contrast medium into the aorta is itself a fine achievement. Rendering the abdominal vessels opaque to X-rays opened new fields for clinical investigation and treatment. The work of these three eminent doctors deserves the applause of all who are interested in the progress of science which is our concern.

When interpreting the arteriograms, he thought he could see arteries and veins and he wanted to call the attention of his colleagues to this point.

The opaque substance passes through the capillaries without losing the property of being radio-opaque unless it comes into contact with a large volume of blood which dilutes the iodide.

During his first investigations in dogs he injected 100% solutions of strontium bromide and lithium bromide (the first radio-opaque substances to be used) into the internal carotid artery and he noted that the veins became opaque as the blood returned from the head. He showed some X-ray plates which confirmed this.

The intra-arterial route for giving treatment was going to be very important and his colleagues had made an original and first-class contribution to its progress and development.

One of his own patients who was suffering from intracranial hypertension (probably caused by serious meningitis) was improved by intracranial injections of sodium iodide. Although he was nearly blind when he was admitted to the Neurology Department, he was now in good health and his vision was nearly normal two years after this treatment.

He wanted to point out, while on the subject of the advantages of intra-arterial drugs, that intra-carotid sodium iodide had brought about permanent or transient improvement in 20% of patients with cranial hypertension. This had not happened after repeated intravenous injections of high doses.

He finished by congratulating Dr. Silva Carvalho on being chairman at such a remarkable meeting; as an eminent man in the profession and as a Portuguese he should be well aware of this.

Mr. Cancella d'Abreu pointed out that the work presented marked an important stage in the progress of medicine by reason of the definite nature of the results and the enormous field which it opened for diagnosis and treatment.

Referring to the use of the arterial route in the treatment of disorders of the limbs, he felt that the small operation to dissect out the artery — the technique used by the authors, according to their recent presentation — was unnecessary. He was sure that the brachial artery at least could be reached percutaneously relatively easily at the elbow in most people. He felt that the same technique could be used in the more superficial parts of all the arteries of the limbs.

He based this assertion on personal experience with the brachial artery. On 15th November 1928 he started to treat a patient with bilateral syphilitic lesions of his palms with intra-arterial 10% sodium iodide. He intended to follow this with a mercurial compound which was only slightly irritating. He used this technique on one side only and compared the progress of the similar lesions because he wanted to carry out a clinical trial of the extent of the local action of the drug when given by this route. His technique was shown to be safe but he was unable to follow it up. Later, however, he had performed brachial puncture on several other patients in order to carry out certain investigations.

He mentioned his experience of this small matter to show that some arterial injections can be carried out by all doctors who are skilled at venepuncture.

He thought highly of the work which had been presented and he was of the opinion that he should take the opportunity of thanking Messrs. Reynaldo dos Santos, Lamas and Caldas for providing the opportunity for increasing the clinical applications of this therapeutic technique, which should be taken up.

Mr. Silvio Rebelo congratulated the speaker and the Society of Medical Science in the presence of which he had presented the results of his very interesting investigations. Turning to the differences in the activity of drugs when they are given intravenously or into an artery, he was of the opinion that the greater safety of the arterial route could not be assumed a priori. When it is given into an artery in a limb and the venous return of that limb is stopped or reduced by an elastic tourniquet, a drug arrives at the cells and acts on them in a concentration which would be dangerous if given by any other route. This maximal effect in an area is readily understandable for it is brought about by the concentration of the drug in the arterioles. However, as far as general effects are concerned, an intra-arterial administration is equivalent to a slow intravenous injection beyond the capillaries. The "concentration" factor is more important than the "quantity" factor in both the therapeutic activities and other actions of drugs.

On the subject of renal arteriography which was mentioned by the speaker, he recalled his work which had been carried out in collaboration with Mr. Celestino da Costa and presented at the Portuguese Society for Biology in 1923. He was of the opinion that this work had demonstrated an inconsistency in the fat-fixing and fat-digesting functions of the lung which had been accepted by Roger and his colleagues. Fats stained with Sudan stain or Scharlach R are held up in the first capillary network which they meet. This is in the lung or the kidney depending whether the route of administration was intravenous or intra-arterial. In their investigations Celestino da Costa and Silvio Rebelo had used the left ventricle for intra-arterial injections.

FIRST COMMUNICATION ON ANGIOPNEUMOGRAPHY

Lopo de Carvalho

(Visualisation, by means of X-rays, of the pulmonary vessels, obtained by injection of an opaque liquid into the right auricle).
Academia das Ciencias de Lisboa, III, 1931.

Summary of the Report of Permanent Member Senhor Egas Moniz to the Division of Sciences at February 19, 1931, Session.

Egas Moniz has read his paper, which was announced, on *Visualisation, by means of X-rays, of the pulmonary vessels obtained by injection of an opaque liquid into the right auricle.*

He, Almeida Lima and I began our work on animals by injections of sodium iodide into the right ventricle, the auricle, and the jugular vein, so obtaining visualisation of the pulmonary arteries and veins. We were afraid that these vessels might be concealed beneath a dark patch due to the passage of the opaque fluid through the abundant capillary network of the lungs, but the radiograms showed that these fears were unfounded. These experiments were carried out on rabbits, dogs, and monkeys, and Egas Moniz has exhibited a number of interesting radiograms. One of these showed not only the pulmonary vascular network but also the hepatic and splenic veins, as a result of entry of the solution into the inferior vena cava.

We next injected the opaque liquid into the arm veins in man, at first on one side only, but then on both sides at the same time. The opaque solutions could be followed on the radiograms as far as the subclavian vein, but visualisation stopped there suddenly.

It was therefore necessary to approach the pulmonary region more closely, and to do that we utilised the external jugular and anterior jugular veins, as we were convinced that by this route the opaque fluid would reach the heart more easily.

Two important findings were made during these studies. The first was that the veins of the neck were not painful when sodium iodide was injected in high concentration. In the arm veins, injections of sodium iodide in concentrations higher than 30 per cent are quite painful, whereas solutions of up to 60 per cent can be injected into the veins of the neck without causing pain. As was found later, the large venous trunks enjoy the same immunity. This difference in sensitivity of the veins of the neck and the limbs, which seems to have been unknown hitherto, made these experiments much easier to carry out.

In the second place, we observed that when very concentrated solutions of sodium iodide were injected into the external jugular vein or even into the subclavian vein, the fluid did not take the natural course of the blood towards the heart, but flowed back in the opposite direction, and this led us to study the mechanism of the venous circulation of the neck, which Egas Moniz has long considered important. The external and anterior jugular veins, which were once considered of no importance, play a notable part in the venous circulation of the neck and brain. In short, we concluded that the two jugular systems, deep and superficial, which are definitely separate only in man, do a great work in ensuring that the blood irrigating the brain has the greatest freedom of return.

We next introduced a tube into the superficial veins of the neck, in order to reach the right ventricle, but did not suceed because of the differing ways in which the external jugular vein opened into the subclavian vein.

It was at this time that we became aware of the work by Forssmann, who successfully introduced a tube as far as the right auricle via an arm vein, and we had recourse to this useful expedient, using tubes which were opaque to X-rays employed for catheterisation of the ureters.

But what concentration of sodium iodide solution could be introduced directly into the right auricle without risk to the patient?

At each systole the heart sends about 100 c.c. of blood towards the lungs. Experiments on the opacity of sodium iodide showed that only with concentrations reaching betwen 2 and 3 per cent did the solution become definitely opaque. As the pulmonary vessels are normally seen faintly in radiograms of the chest, it might be suficient to use low concentrations to obtain an increase in visualisation, so giving rise to satisfactory angiograms of the lungs.

It was already known that 60 per cent sodium iodide solutions could be injected into the veins of the neck without adverse effect. Nonetheless, preliminary experiments had to be carried out before a high concentration of sodium iodide was taken as far as the heart, in order to determine whether or not such high concentrations, in contact with a mass of blood, would dissolve (mix) rapidly.

A few cubic centimetres of iodide solutions were poured into glass vessels containing blood. Radiographic exposures obtained at that very moment showed that solution occurred immediately. Egas Moniz has shown interesting films of these experiments.

It was only after this that increasing amounts of iodide solution were injected into the right auricle in man so as to obtain visualisation of the pulmonary vessels.

The radiograms obtained before and after the injection, and presented by Egas Moniz, show an enormous difference. The large vessels, which are barely outlined in ordinary radiograms of the lungs, become definitely visible and their ramifications can be followed right down to the finest branches. It is as if the imperfectly visualised outline of the vessels in ordinary radiograms of the lungs has added to it a reinforcing effect on all the vessels from the injection of sodium iodide into the auricle, so that their prolongations and subdivisions are completed.

Successful angiopneumography having been obtained in normal individuals, it remained to define the advantages which would result clinically. Only experience and continuation of the work which has been started will provide an answer to this, but at the moment its value can be foreseen in the differential diagnosis of vascular tumours and cysts of the lung and, probably, in certain cases of pulmonary tuberculosis. Certain details have already been observed, but nothing can be stated with any assurance at the moment. In physiological investigations, introduction of a tube as far as the auricle and into the vena cava, which is also accessible by this means, can bring new understanding. Local treatment of pulmonary diseases with large amounts of solutions of drugs which are easily soluble in blood could also be tried, using a procedure similar to that which has enabled us to obtain pneumograms.

These are suggestions and prospects for further work, which the results obtained in these preliminary experiments justify in some way, but only experience, in the biological field, can throw light on these important problems.

For the present, one single finding has been made, and there is no doubt about its importance: this is that angiopneumography, or more simply pneumography, can be carried out without risk to the patient.

SECOND COMMUNICATION ON ANGIOPNEUMOGRAPHY

Egas Moniz, Lopo de Carvalho and Almeida Lima
Lisbon

(Angiopneumographie, Presse Méd. (Paris), 39(53): 996-999 (July 4) 1931.)
Translated from French by Robert E. Asnis, Ph.D., Philadelphia.

We have been trying for some time to obtain a visualization of the pulmonary arteries, or rather of the blood vesels (arteries and veins) of the lungs, which would justify an article with the above title. The arteries and veins of the lungs run beside the bronchi. Both correspond for the most part in their branchings to the divisions of the bronchial tree. Our desire to develop a technique for angiopneumography was based on clinical considerations, and we were especially interested in it as a possible aid in the diagnosis of neoplasms of the lungs. It was also felt that it might make possible a more precise diagnosis of pulmonary tuberculosis, although this consideration was not of such great importance to us, since the diagnosis of the latter disease is now being accomplished quite satisfactorily by procedures for clinical examinations which are already at our disposal.

In the differential diagnosis of vascularized tumours and of cysts, for example, a visualization of the circulation of the former would afford us a new diagnostic tool. A similar method has made possible the differential diagnosis in the brain of highly vascularized tumours, as distinguished from others which have no appreciable circulation.

But the problem of visualization of the vessels of the lungs presented great difficulties. We had to use a fluid which was both opaque to X-rays and harmless in its passage through the lungs. Furthermore, it was necessary to introduce this fluid into the venous circulation, in order for it to make the circuit from the right heart to the left heart via the lungs. And the large amount of circulating blood in the ventricle of the adult would necessarily reduce the concentration of the intravenously injected opaque solution to a percentage which could not be seen with X-rays. This was the greatest difficulty to be overcome.

Another problem also occurred to us. In view of the high degree of vascularization of the lungs, any opaque fluid introduced into them would produce, instead of a visible circulatory system, simply an opaque spot, such as we had already observed in several peripheral circulatory systems. If such were the case, one would see only the great vessels and our investigation would be almost useless. In order to obtain a clear preliminary idea of what would happen, we performed our first experiments in animals.

As the opaque fluids we chose solutions of sodium iodide, which had already been studied by two of us from the three aspects of their toxicity, their irritant effects on the tissues and their opacity to X-rays[1].

1) Egas Moniz: Diagnostic des tumeurs cérébrales et épreuve de l'encephalographie artérielle, Paris, Masson et Cie, 1931, p.239 ff.

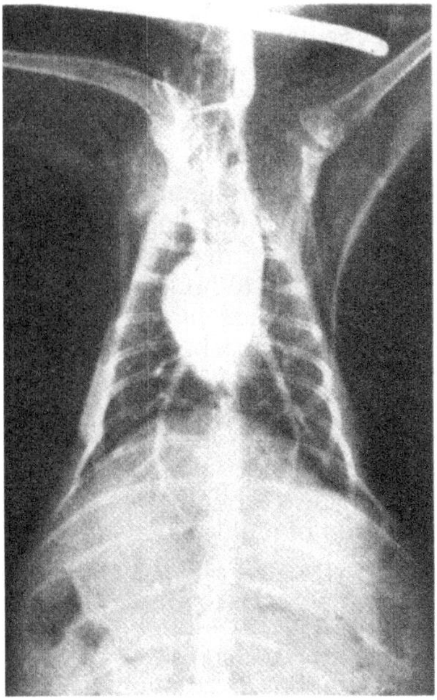

Fig 1: Arteriopneumogram of a rabbit. Injection into the jugular vein of a 40 per cent of sodium iodide.

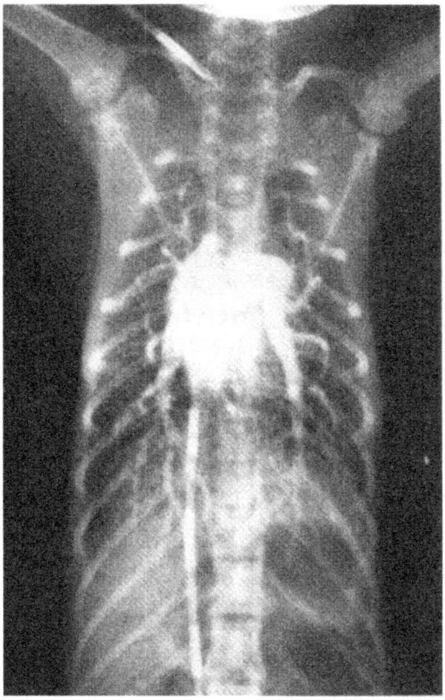

Fig 2: Arteriopneumogram of a monkey. Injection of an 80 per cent solution of sodium iodide into the right auricle by catheterization of the inferior vena cava.

The first animal chosen for the experiments was the rabbit. We injected a 40% sodium iodide solution directly into the right ventricle, this being very easy to accomplish at the level of the 4th intercostal space, and we later tried injecting it into the jugular vein (Fig. 1). The pulmonary vessels were thereby outlined to the extent that they resembled a visualized bronchial tree.

In order to obtain more perfect outlines the concentration of the sodium iodide solution was increased to 80%. Figure 1 shows the radiographic appearance of the lungs after injection into the jugular vein of a 40% solution. The amounts injected were 5 cc or more.

We also produced good visualization of the pulmonary network in the dog by means of large injections of a 100% solution of sodium iodide into the jugular vein.

In the monkey (Fig. 2)[2] it was also possible to obtain beautiful angiopneumograms.

It was after repeated experiments of this sort in animals that we decided to begin experiments in man.

We first made injections of a 25% sodium iodide solution as rapidly as possible into an arm vein, and reduced the venous return of blood at the moment of injection by the application of elastic ligatures to the thighs and the uninjected arm and by the application of pressure to the internal jugular veins. We were then able to follow, by means of radiographs, the course of the opaque fluid up to the subclavian vein, but at this point the opacity suddenly disappeared.

We later made simultaneous injections into the veins of both arms, and we even increased the concentration of the sodium iodide up to 30%, which is the upper limit for painless injections, but the radiographs of the thorax still remained negative.

It was therefore necessary to increase the percentage of iodide in the solutions used and to inject them as near as possible to the right ventricle, in order to avoid loss of the needed concentration in the large mass of blood.

The right ventricle of an adult human has a capacity of 170 cc but the systolic output must be approximately 100 cc[3] according to the experiments of Henderson and Prince, Meakins and Davis, Dautreband, etc.

In each cardiac cycle (for a period of less than one second), we therefore had to get into the right ventricle an amount of sodium iodide which would still retain its opacity in this amount of blood.

From these facts we could readily calculate the impossibility of achieving our purpose by injections into the arm veins. But if one could succeed in injecting quickly a sufficiently concentrated iodide solution into the superior vena cava, for example, one might just possibly have a chance of visualizing the pulmonary vessels.

Could these foreseeable possibilities be tested in any way except by further experimentation?

We had tested in animals the effects of sodium iodide on the lungs and had demonstrated that concentrations of 50% to 100% were well tolerated. But that did not justify our injecting such high

2) This angiopneumogram was obtained by an injection into the right auricle. The catheter was introduced via the inferior vena cava.

3) On the basis of these experiments we are convinced that the output should in general be lower and that it is probably 50 to 70 cc.

percentages into the large vessels of the neck or thorax of a human subject. We therefore began the cautious administration of progressively increasing doses in man. But now a new difficulty arose.

The Insensitivity of the Veins and of the Large Venous Trunks of the Neck. — We considered puncturing the large veins of the neck. Some experiments made on cadavers convinced us that it was very easy to reach both the brachio-cephalic trunk and the superior vena cava. By introducing a needle toward the right between the sternal and clavicular parts of the sterno-cleido-mastoid behind the sternum, one at once encounters the brachio-cephalic trunk and the superior vena cava. These results encouraged us to attempt the same procedure in a living subject.

We have performed a fairly large series of experiments for the purpose of introducing the needle into the internal jugular, the subclavian, the brachio-cephalic and the superior vena cava. The needle was certainly introduced into these veins; but we only very rarely succeeded in obtaining any blood by aspiration of the syringe. And in order to inject an iodide solution *it was necessary to be absolutely certain that the needle had entered one of these large vessels. An injection, which was made outside of the vein, could cause serious harm.* It was essential to know that the needle was well introduced and *that it could not spring out during the injection.*

This difficulty of the uncertainty of being in one of the large venous trunks of the neck was the result of their low internal pressure.

The blood did not enter the syringe even on aspiration.

In the superior vena cava and in brachio-cephalic trunks the pressure is actually negative.

Although we used a quite powerful electric aspirator and needles which were one millimeter in diameter, we rarely succeeded in obtaining blood, especially from the sub-clavian veins. We had already at that time attempted by certain other procedures, which we shall here only mention very briefly, and without any danger or pain for the patients, the injection of more concentrated iodide solutions into other veins of the neck. The concentrations had been raised to as high as 50% and 60% sodium iodide. In one of our experiments we injected 16 cc of a 60% solution into the subclavian vein of a patient. At the time when this amount had been injected, the patient complained, and we stopped the injection. He had experienced a very violent but transitory pain in the neck. Two hours later he felt entirely well. A radiograph showed an opaque spot at the level of the external third of the clavicle. A marked venous distention and an extravasation of some of the fluid had occurred. A radiograph taken several minutes later showed the spot to have become less opaque. Another made the next day showed no trace of the spot. A very careful examination of these radiographs revealed that the fluid did not advance, at least not entirely, in the direction of the bloodstream toward the superior vena cava. A large part of the injected fluid flowed back in the opposite direction toward the external portion of the subclavian vein. This vein had been dilated, and at the end of the injection an extravasation of the fluid had occurred. Fortunately, this had been harmless, since the patient had complained of pain, and the injection had been stopped at once.

We also introduced directly, either into the external jugular or the internal jugular vein, solutions of 35%, 40%, 45%, 50%, 55%, and 60%, sodium iodide. *There was never any pain; but the liquid did not descend en masse. A part of it ascended in the vein.*

The insensitivity of the veins of the neck to injections of sodium iodide at percentages which were quite painful when injected into the veins of the limbs revealed a great difference between the sensitivities of these two classes of veins. That has been a favourable factor, which has facilitated our experiments.

We then attempted the catheterization of certain neck veins, such as the external and anterior jugular veins, the loss of whose functioning does not have serious consequences. Ordinary ureteral catheters were used. All of the manipulations involved were well tolerated without any inconvenience to the patients. But we only succeeded in reaching the subclavian vein on two occasions. The catheter, due especially to the diverging arrangement of the external jugular veins (the right one particularly), followed a course external to the subclavian vein. In one of our films the tip of the catheter could be seen in the subclavian vein, but not all of the injected fluid followed the course of the blood toward the superior vena cava. A part of it certainly flowed in the desired direction, but another and probably larger part stopped or flowed in a retrograde direction.

The Mechanism of the Venous Circulation of the Neck. — All of these findings led us to a consideration of the mechanism of the circulation of the neck and of the disturbances in the hydraulics of the venous network which are caused by the introduction of a fluid having a density different from that of the blood.

With regard to the physiology of the venous circulation of the neck, it should be noted that the most dependable circulation is that which runs from the brain via the internal jugulars. The circulation of the subclavian veins is always slowed when there is an increased outflow of blood from the brain.

Indeed this fact might be expected on the basis of more central anatomic disposition of the internal jugulars and their more direct course in relation to the superior vena cava. There is, however, another feature of the anatomic disposition which must certainly be of importance in the mechanism of the venous circulation of the neck. The schematic drawing in Fig. 3 shows that the external jugular enters the subclavian vein at an acute angle running in a direction away from the internal jugular. The external jugular forms several anastomoses with the internal jugular and with the anterior jugular [4], which is in general less important. The superficial jugulars drain the blood from the walls and surrounding tissues of the skull.

Fig. 3: I, internal jugular vein; II, external jugular vein; III subclavian vein; IV, superior vena cava. We have not shown the anterior jugular vein in order to avoid complicating the diagram.

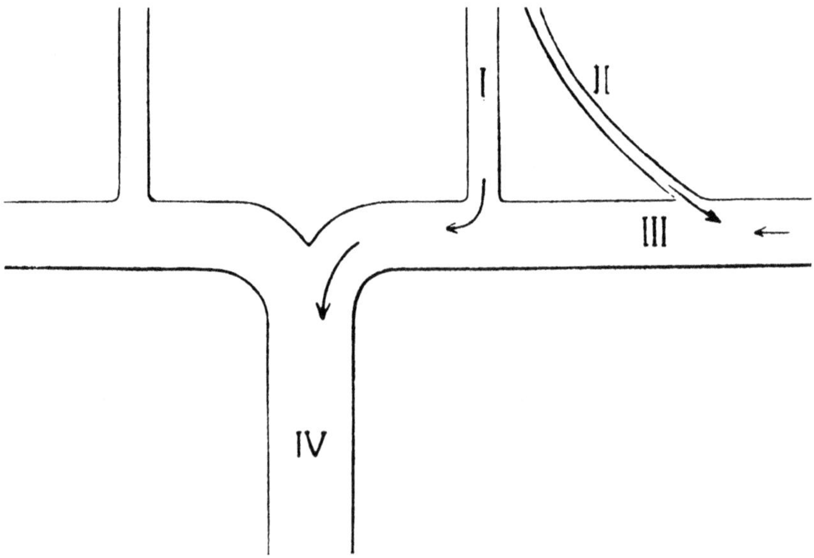

4 We have not represented this vein in the schematic drawing in order to avoid complications. When the anterior jugulars have a certain volume, this volume is inversely proportional to that in the external jugulars. The anterior jugulars often have an oblique disposition similar to that which is shown in the schematic drawing for the external jugulars.

When the flow of blood to the brain from the carotids is very strong both the deep and superficial jugular systems, which assure the drainage of the blood from the entire head, are very full of blood. The current of the blood in the external jugular runs in direction opposed to that of the blood in the subclavian vein which flows toward the heart (Fig. 3-III). In our opinion this constitutes an anatomic-physiologic protective mechanism which serves to facilitate the flow of blood from the internal jugular into the superior vena cava.

When we tried to inject the iodide solutions into the subclavian or the external or anterior jugular vein, a large part of the injected fluid always flowed backward in a direction opposed to that of the current of the blood. This was a result of the special mechanics of the venous circulation of the region involved.

In addition, the entrance into the circulation of a fluid of higher density than that of the blood must have produced disturbances in the hydraulics of these collectors of venous blood. However, the importance of this factor has been difficult for us to determine owing to a lack of precise data.

What must be noted is the fact that injections via the subclavian vein do not flow with the desired speed toward the heart.

This fact is of physiologic interest, but it has been a serious hindrance to the carrying out of our experiments. Indeed, it made necessary the direct injection of the opaque fluid into the vena cava or into the auricle. But these regions could not be reached by catheterization of the superficial veins of the neck. A surgical operation would not have been justified, and angiopneumography requiring such an operation would be of no clinical interest.

Among all of the radiographs obtained in human subjects in these first experiments, there were at least two or three in which the outlines of the pulmonary vessels seemed to us to be more distinct after the injection of certain solutions of sodium iodide. This encouraged us to continue our experimentation.

Direct Injections into the Auricle. — At about this time we learned that Forssmann had succeeded in reaching the auricle with a catheter introduced via one of the veins in the fold of the elbow without any difficulties. We then adopted this route and thereby achieved positive results.

Our experiments in animals were first resumed. A description of all of our animal experiments is beyond the scope of this article. It will suffice, we believe, to publish two of the radiographs which we obtained. That shown in Fig. 4 was made after an injection via a

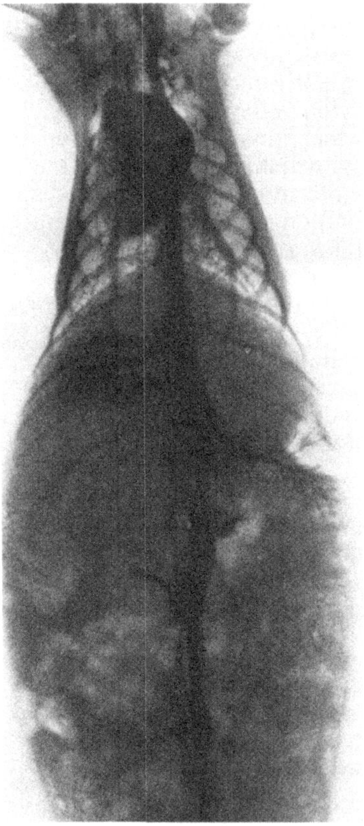

Fig. 4: A forced injection into the right auricle of a rabbit's heart. A part of the opaque fluid has passed down into the inferior vena cava and into the hepatic veins.

Fig. 5: Introduction of the catheter via the jugular vein into the right auricle and into the inferior vena cava. The hepatic veins and the splenic vein are visible.

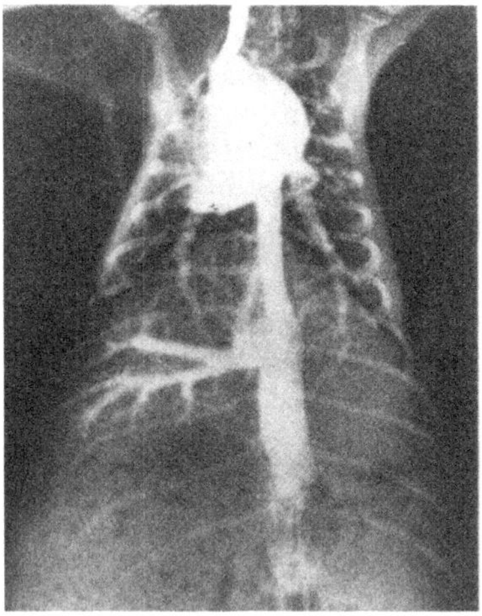

catheter into the right auricle of a rabbit. The injection was made under considerable pressure. The angiopneumogram is quite distinct. The excess fluid has flowed into the inferior vena cava and the hepatic veins. In the radiograph shown in Fig. 5 the catheter, which was introduced into the auricle, has passed down into the inferior vena cava. Here the angiopneumogram is less distinct than in the preceding radiograph and there is a visualization of the venous systems of the liver and spleen.

These two experiments explain a fact which Forssmann [5] has

5) Werner Forssmann: Die Sondierung des rechten Herzens. Klinische Wochenschrift, November 5, 1929.

reported in his article. He there asks why the catheter in a patient entered the inferior vena cava rather than the right ventricle as it had done in a cadaver. This was because the auriculo-ventricular valve in the living subject prevents the entrance of the catheter into the ventricle, and therefore, if one pushes the catheter too far, it very easily reaches the opening of the inferior vena cava and very easily passes beyond it, if there is an insufficiency of Eustache's valve. This illustrates the fact that at the moment of the introduction of the catheter into the auricle one must be careful not to force it.

These results have given us the idea of obtaining visualizations of some of the systems arising from the inferior vena cava, such as, for example, the hepatic venous system. But we believe that such procedures might be dangerous.

After these experiments in animals, we resumed our work with human subjects, and the first human angiopneumograms were obtained by the following technique: The introduction of a catheter into a vein can be made in two ways: either with a small trocar, through the lumen of which a catheter can be introduced; or by what seemed to us to be the simpler procedure (especially when the veins are not very large) of making a small incision in the vein through which the catheter could be inserted.

In our first experiments we used 70cm ureteral catheters, which were radiopaque and the olivary tips of which had been cut off. We have found them quite satisfactory. More recently, we have been using special radiopaque cardiac catheters [6], which afford a better delivery of fluid. For the intra-auricular injection we use one syringe containing 2 cc of physiologic saline and another containing 10 cc of an 80% or 120% aqueous solution of chemically pure sodium iodide.

Preparation of the Patient. — The injection must be made with the patient in the fasting state; and he should be seated. It is easier to use the left side because of the anatomic disposition of the external and internal jugular veins, which is in general more favourable for the introduction of a catheter on that side. The procedure is exactly like that for a simple intravenous injection and the forearm is wrapped in a sterile towel. The vein is punctured, and a ureteral type catheter, which is radiopaque, and which has just been passed through a 10% sodium citrate solution is introduced. An assistant takes the other end of the catheter, to which is attached a syringe containing physiologic saline, and the saline is slowly injected during the introduction of the catheter.

6) P. Gentle & Co., 49 rue Saint-André-des Arts, Paris.

This whole procedure is carried out with the aid of a fluoroscope. In the external portion of the subclavian vein the catheter tends to pass into the external jugular. By raising the patient's arm when the catheter does not follow the desired path and by aiding its progress with the fingers in the clavicular region, where the catheter can be felt, the right auricle can easily be reached.If one attempts to push the catheter further, it may, as we have previously noted, enter the inferior vena cava.

Since it was thought to be necessary to reduce to a minimum the blood in the heart in order to prevent the percentage of iodide from being lowered below the limit required for opacity, we decided, at the moment of injection, to constrict with tourniquets both of the thighs, the free arm and the neck. An assistant exerted pressure with his fist on the inferior vena cava, and another assistant exerted pressure on the internal jugulars, since the pressure of the neck tourniquet was always inadequate. All of this took about ten seconds.

Other radiographs of the pulmonary vessels were made without taking these precautions, and they always turned out well. We have therefore abandoned the above-described original practice.

The apparatus having been placed in position for the radiography, the liquid is injected. It suffices to inject 5 to 6 cc of a 120% iodide solution as quickly as possible. The discharge of the contents of the ampoule must be made when the syringe still contains 1 to 2 cc of saline, the injection of which is continued. The patient does not experience any discomfort. Sometimes there is a marked but indefinable sensation of taste and slight transitory cough.

When the radiography has been completed a syringe containing saline is again attached to the catheter, saline is injected to expel the remaining iodide solution, and the catheter is then withdrawn.

The Radiographs. — Radiographs of the thorax always show some vessels which are close to the bronchial tree. One might expect to see the bronchi, but these are generally permeable to X-rays. Only the blood in the vessels is slightly opaque, and if they are sclerosed, their visibility is increased. The injection of the sodiium iodide solution into the auricle increases the visibility of the more or less well-outlined vessels seen in the normal radiograph. One which follow the same course, are visible. Up to the present time we have found it impossible to distinguish these from one another in the angiopneumograms.

We are at present engaged in the preparation of stereoscopic angiopneumograms.

It seems to us that the solutions of sodium iodide which we

have used were quite satisfactory. However, now that the technique has been worked out, some more concentrated sodium iodide solutions [7], as well as other kinds of opaque fluids will be tried.

We believe that the condition of the patient should determine the percentage of iodide to be used. Thus in tubercular patients it is necessary to adjust the percentage according to the condition of their lungs.

In these first experiments we were not interested in the pathologic cases to which the method can be applied. Such a study will constitute the second step in our investigations.

In one of our cases we noted in an otherwise normal radiograph a small spot which could have been interpreted either as a calcified nodule or as a vessel. The angiopneumography did not increase the visibility of this spot. It was certainly a calcified nodule. We have verified the opposite kind of picture in some of our cases in which vessels perpendicular to the plane of the radiograph produced spots even in simple radiographies. In the angiopneumograms these spots became denser.

The angiopneumography as we are now obtaining it, without any discomfort for the patient, and by a very simple method, is already an accomplished fact, which seemed to us of sufficient interest to make known, even before making a study of its advantages in clinical practice.

These catheterizations which can be extended as far as the inferior vena cava will help in clarifying certain physiologic problems.

The injection into the right auricle, without danger, of solutions which are highly concentrated, but which are rapidly diluted by the blood [8], also offers the hope of an improved therapeutic technique for pulmonary diseases. Thus one should be able by this method to achieve local medication, since the concentrated solutions needed for this purpose would immediately afterwards be rapidly diluted by the blood.

We are here only offering some suggestions for future investigations. Our first findings permit us to foresee their possibility.

In concluding we wish to repeat that we have fortunately never had any difficulties with this procedure in any of our patients.

We would like to thank the Rocha Cabral Institute of Lisbon and the Board of National Education for the assistance which they have given us.

7) We have not been able to obtain solutions of this kind which are of sufficiently good quality to be used for such purposes.

8) Before injecting these high percentages of sodium iodide into the auricle, we carried out some radiographic experiments with blood in vitro. These showed the dilution of the concentrated iodide solution to be instantaneous.

FIRST COMMUNICATION ON LYMPHOGRAPHY

Hernâni Monteiro

(Radiographic demonstration of the lymphatic system in the living, with the collaboration of Roberto de Carvalho, Alvaro Rodrigues, and Sousa Pereira). Annales d'Anatomie Pathologique et d'Anatomie Normale, **8**, 1931, Meeting of 5th February, 1931.

Although for a long time the morphological study of the lymphatic system has deserved attention from anatomists, it still remains to-day a field open to investigation, and some present-day workers have carried out studies of real value.

Using mercury, Prussian blue (Gerota's method), and other procedures, anatomists have been solely concerned with determining the morphology and topography of the lymphatic network in cadavers. However, even though such studies may be of great interest, particularly from the anatomical point of view, another problem - and one which is no less interesting and could even have the most important consequences - occurs to us at the present time: that of demonstrating the lymphatic system radiographically in the living.

Inspired by the brilliant work carried out in Lisbon on arteriography by Egas Moniz and Reynaldo dos Santos, we had the idea of trying to visualise the lymphatic system in the living by means of a radiographic method.

Acquaintance with the technique of injecting the lymphatics by Gerota's method - acquaintance which Alvaro Rodrigues and A. de Sousa Pereira [1] had gained in Paris under Professor Rouvière, - facilitated the performance of these investigations.

For the success of our studies, it was essential to find a liquid which would give a good radiographic image and would pass through the fine needles that we used, and then to spread into the lymph vessels, and at the same time have no toxic or irritant action which would be harmful to the patient.

After many experiments on dogs, starting in November of last year and using various products containing salts of elements with a high atomic weight, we succeeded in obtaining radiographic pictures of the lymph vessels of living animals by injecting into the inguinal glands and the glands of the neck [2].

Figure 1 shows one radiogram obtained during some of these experiments. None of the animals in which we injected the lymphatics, and whose radiograms we now present, had any post-operative disturbances.

As our research is in progress, with the aim of carrying out radiographic studies on the lymphatics in man and of demonstrating their clinical applications, we were not considering presenting the results obtained so far until a later stage. However, recently we received a paper from Professor Funaoka in Kyoto, referring to the

Fig. 1. The First lymphography in dog.

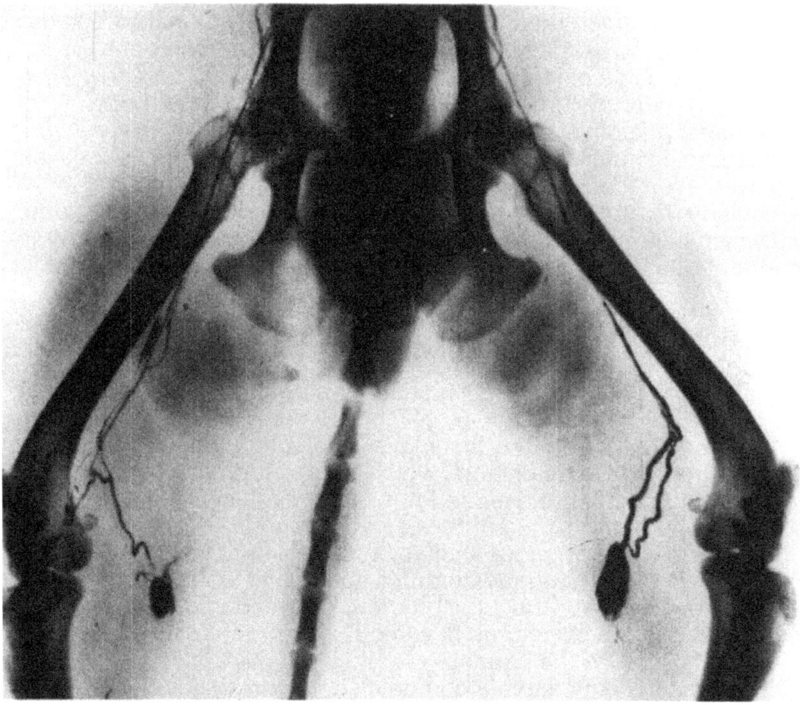

same problem[3] , we decided to present the results we achieved in some of our experiments in this preliminary note to the Société Anatomique.

In a subsequent paper, we shall publish in detail the technique used for the injections and we will indicate the opaque substances employed and the results obtained.

(Work carried out at the Experimental Surgery Laboratory of Oporto Faculty of Medicine, with a grant from the National Education Board and from Dr. Roberto Carvalho's Radiological Clinic.)

1) Alvaro Rodrigues and J. Sousa Pereira: on the large lymphatic trunks at the base of the neck. Annal. d'Anat. pathol. et d'Anat. normale médico-chirurgicàle, 7th year, No.8, 1930.

2) Our investigations were carried out on dogs under general anaesthesia, either with Somnifen-morphine or with alcohol.

3) Reports from department 3 of the Anatomical Institute of the Imperial University, Kyoto, issued by Prof. Seigo Funaoka (Head of the Department), Series D. Investigations on the Physiology of Lymph Movements Vol. 1 Radiography of the lymph vessels. Kyoto, 1930.

FIRST COMMUNICATION ON DIRECT PHLEBOGRAPHY

João Cid dos Santos

(Direct phlebography. The idea. Technique. Preliminary results).
Journal International de Chirurgie, 1938.

The concept of rendering the venous system radio-opaque was carried in effect a long time ago. The use of solutions known to be opaque to X-rays on intravenous injection, inevitably led to venography. But the first realisation of this objective in living humans by Berberich and Hirsch 15 years ago was rather original as it ushered in the era of urography.

A problem, however, cannot always be completely tackled in the right way from the outset. It is the misfortunes but also the "glory" of their pioneers which remain associated with an idea. Berberich and Hirsch were the first to carry out arteriography and phlebography in living humans. The pictures were small, incomplete, and poorly visualised, but the possibilities of the method had been demonstrated. Now, whereas phlebography has hardly developed at all, for various reasons, arteriography has made great progress, as is known, in the hands of Reynaldo dos Santos and Egas Moniz.

If we consider present knowledge of arteriography and compare it with that existing ten or twelve years ago, we are amazed at the distance we have come. It must be recognised that, as a result of the work carried out, we speak to-day of the arterial circulation from a basis of knowledge which was non-existent a short time ago. The newer vasographic problems can now be approached in quite a different spirit.

Even if phlebography gave way to the development of arteriography, it was nonetheless studied from time to time. The current use of opaque solutions in excretion urography and the results of arteriography constantly drew attention to the veins.

Free-flush phlebograms were obtained by Demel, Sgalitzer and Kollert (1931), whose detailed study of normal and pathological veins, and in particular their valvular aspects, were of undoubted interest; it was the same workers who, in 1934, published the first two phlebograms of thrombosis of the subclavian vein. In 1932, Wohleben had obtained radiograms of several normal upper limbs after injection of a solution intended for urography, and, in 1935, Veal and McFertridge published two more phlebograms of thrombosis of the subclavian vein.

In another area, we find that Saito (1930) injected an iodide solution into a vein after applying two tourniquets, above and below the site of puncture, and in this way visualising several cases of varices. The principal phlebographic studies, however, in the field of varices are undoubtedly those of Barber and Orley (1932), followed by those of Patey, Tatham and Nicholas (1933) and, in America, those of Pomeranz and Tunick. It was to those workers that a more profound radiographic study of areas of varicosity was due, although Demel and Sgalitzer had already mentioned it, and it was, I think, Pomeranz and Tunick who for the first time suggested the use of opaque solutions, even with the aim of sclerosing the varicose veins.

Finally, in 1935, Reynaldo dos Santos, published the first phlebogram of the vena cava (suture), obtained by my method and I myself have in press a case of venous spasm of the upper limb (Rev. de Chir.). I have not yet been able to procure the articles by a number of workers, such as Allen and Barker, Ratschow, Adamek and Friedländer, etc., who have also investigated direct phlebography in man. But this short summary is not intended to be a history of phlebography.

However, the essential problems of phlebography remained unsolved. To get to know the phlebographic appearance of a normal or pathological vein is undoubtedly important, but this appearance should be set within the framework of the venous circulation, for the problem of phlebography is in reality much wider: *it is the anatomical and physiological aspects of the venous circulation which we must get to know in the first place, and then the pathological, anatomical and physiological aspects of the same circulation.* Only then will the isolated pictures of veins assume their true value. This is what concerned me when, on the prompting advice of Reynaldo dos Santos, I undertook my research on phlebography.

My labours were greatly simplified by all the previous work on arteriography which, while still a medical student, I had seen coming into being in our Department. I was present at the first translumbar puncture of the aorta and I followed step by step the slow evolution of this new diagnostic method. This experience helped me to avoid many pitfalls.

Even if the basic concepts behind the two methods are similar to one another, however, that is where their similarities cease. The problems from the point of view of carrying out the actual procedure in phlebography are the reverse of those of arteriography.

As time went on we came to realise to-day that the major technical problem in arteriography was always essentially one of chemistry - the contrast medium. All the persistent difficulties arose, and still arise, from it. The biochemical properties of the solutions used had to be adapted to the conditions of the examination to be carried out. As the contrast medium had to pass through a regional capillary network, one had to take into account not only its general toxicity but also, and especially, its local effect on the small vessels and tissues associated with the artery into which the injection was given.

The problem of pain was intimately bound up with this.

This apart, the technique was quite simple, for, with a given flow of blood, - once a mixture with the contrast medium concentrated enough to provide a radiological picture - had been obtained, it was only necessary to maintain the injection for the time required for the first few cc of the opaque mixture to reach the tissues. An exposure made at this time should inevitably reveal the entire picture of the arterial tree, depending on the vessel injected. In arteriography our influence ceases at the point of the needle; thanks to its rapid flow, the arterial blood does the rest; we can hardly interfere.

The problem of technique in phlebography is quite different, for though the arterial tree of each region of our bodies depends on one vessel, the venous tree of each region has its origin dispersed through the tissues themselves. That is to say that true physiological phlebography of each region can only be carried out by means of an injection into the artery upon which the region depends, even if it entails our making the exposure a little later when the opaque substance is already in the veins. This is *arterio-phlebography,* which is certainly useful, and which has not had its last word. But at the moment we do not find it to have the usefulness necessary for a study of the venous system, because during its passage through the tissues, opaque medium remain partly fixed there - this being the basis of all therapy by the arterial route. In addition, the opacity of the veins is slight and sometimes non-existent. For us to envisage the possibility of obtaining good phlebograms by the arterial route, it would entail the solution's use in such concentrations which might be dangerous, and again I do not know if reactions of a spastic nature might not, in spite of everything, prevent the passage through the tissues of sufficient quantities of the solution to visualise the veins completely. This is therefore a question to be considered as a whole.

I therefore investigated whether, by injecting into superficial veins, which are more or less consistently present, I could obtain pictures of the veins of an entire region, which could be compared one with another. *I was thus led to visualisation of the major deep collecting veins by injecting the major superficial colllecting veins.* Thus the external saphenous vein enabled me to visualise the popliteal and femoral veins, while the internal saphenous was the means of access for visualisation of the iliac veins and the inferior vena cava. In the upper limb, the basilic and cephalic veins were chosen for visualisation of the axillary vein or the subclavian vein and the superior vena cava. The preliminary results were encouraging and I continued my study of *direct free-flow phlebograpy.* Normal pictures were very simple, as was easy to foresee; nothing but single venous trunks, if the leg is excepted, where a more or less important network of tributaries of the external saphenous vein was always visualised when the latter was injected behind the malleolus. *This is therefore not the venous counterpart of arteriography, and phlebography as such cannot hope to hold a place equal to that of the other method.*

For the present, the field of application of phlebography is in part limited to lesions of the same large venous trunks as are opacified in normal man. It is something, however, to be able to make a direct study of the early or later pictures of cases of thrombophlebitis and the circulatory disturbances resulting from it. The books are significantly silent on this question. The method, however, also has a physiological value, since it is the free circulation into which the injection is given, and its value is thus increased by the new possibilities of studying the problems of normal and pathological venous dynamics, such as vasomotor actions and various aspects of blood circulation, whether these relate to the routes taken or the rate of blood flow.

Some of these problems were touched upon during the 150 phlebographic examinations I carried out with the aid of my loyal collaborators, David Benoliel, Fernanda P. Ferreira, Almerindo Lessa and Antonio Bugalho.

Elsewhere, the retrograde circulation of varices had been demonstrated by British and American workers, who injected the contrast medium into the upper part of the visible lesions. I myself had been working for some time on the question of intra-arterial injections followed by stasis, and, in connection with these investigations, of which he presented several cases to the Société de Chirurgie, Reynaldo dos Santos reminded me that intravenous injections with stasis by Bier's method could be used for therapeutic purposes. I was thus led to use stasis in association with retrograde injections in cases of varices. The phlebographic pictures were very good, as there was no valve system to prevent the opaque solution from entering the pathological venous tree. The results obtained so far make me believe that *retrograde phlebography with stasis* will rapidly become the method par excellence in the symptomatic study of varices. In association with examination by free-flush phlebography, it will provide anatomical and physio-pathological information on each case which to-day is impossible to obtain by other methods. In addition, phlebography with stasis opens the door to a wide range of therapeutic activity, the basis and results of which I will report later.

This having been said, does the method involve any dangers? Is it harmless to the veins? Can it cause severe reactions? It is essential to know.

Now I believe I can say “no”. In nearly 150 examinations, the majority of patients with diseases of the venous system, I have had no severe reactions to report, and not even one untoward incident. We have behind us the tremendous experience gained in excretion urography. The safety of the current contrast media even when injected very rapidly, is almost complete, from either the local or the general point of view.

As for the danger of phlebography — induced embolism this is not even theoretically possible, for the injected solution could not cause obliteration of the vein or detach the head of a thrombus, because the compulsory slowness of the injections in such cases would never allow it. I shall come back to this starting point.

“Obsessed” by the idea of arteriography which was the starting point of our work, I wanted to follow the same path, but I had to free myself from such ideas and apply myself to using those routes which presented themselves. As it is to-day, unlike arteriography, phlebography is not a method for the general study of symptoms. Its field of action remains confined to the physiology and pathology of veins, in particular phlebitis (and not all cases), varices of whatever origin, and certain problems relating to vasomotor actions and the circulation of the blood.

Nonetheless, that is sufficient, I believe, to justify its use and continued study.

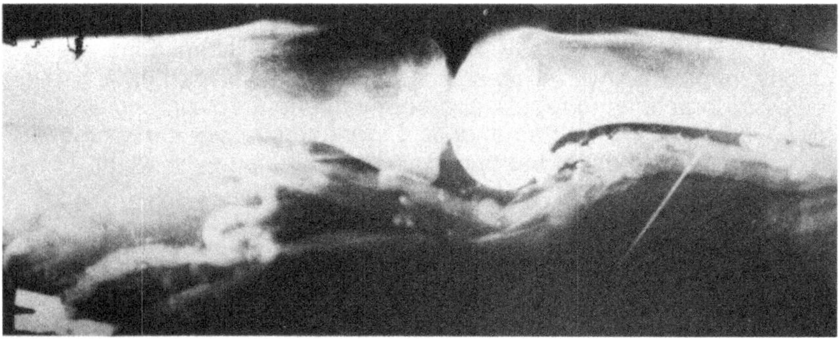

Incompetence of the left saphena parva.
Incompetence of the left internal gastrocnemian vein.

A first demonstrative case. This incompetent internal gastrocnemian vein, should not be taken for the saphena parva.
At mid leg its communication vein became incompetent, perforates the fascia and is followed by superficial varices.
Stereographic vision is excellent.

By kind permission of the Royal College of Surgeons, Edinburgh.

Dos Santos Collection No.5409

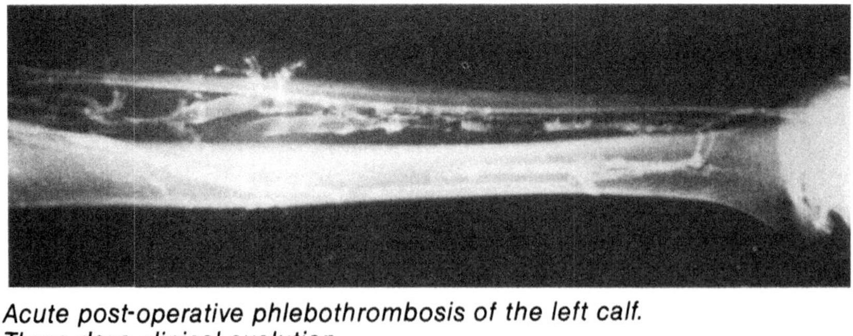

Acute post-operative phlebothrombosis of the left calf.
Three days clinical evolution.

Phlebographic technique:-

Horizontal position. Low malleolar tourniquet. Injection through a superficial vein of the foot. After 40 cc were injected, a second tourniquet is tightened about the knee. 20 cc more are then injected.

Dos Santos Collection No.5747

RADIOGRAPHY

a) *Total phlebography of the limbs* - We are too often obliged to follow existing technical conditions, which were created for a different purpose from our own. Thus, radiological machines were not intended for radiographing an entire limb all at once.

Now *the circulation of a limb should be studied from one end to another. Everything is of interest to us, whether the examination is carried out for the purposes of physiological study or to reveal lesions, for any primary or secondary damage to blood vessels will nearly always have repercussions both upstream and down stream.* This would be sufficient to justify vascular examination of the whole limb, but most times we do not know the actual site of the lesion. It may be found in one segment of the limb when we believe it to be in another.

This is why, from the outset, I radiographed entire limbs by placing two 30 x 40cm frames lengthwise or sometimes, with very large limbs, three frames widthwise.

The importance of this total visualisation was obvious and it became a routine. With my colleague, A. Lamas, I also used it in arteriography.

At present, the details remain to be perfected without introducing too many complications. I do not think it is necessary for special long films to be manufactured. It would be sufficient to have made a frame 30 x 80 cm, in which two 30 x 40 cm films could be placed lengthwise, with intensifying screens of the same measurements. Possibly, a frame 40 x 90 cm which could contain 3 films 30 x 40 cm in size placed widthwise with these intensifying screens could be useful for very long or, especially, very fat limbs.

It goes without saying that the Potter-Bucky diaphragm cannot be used under these conditions, but nonetheless the radiograms are very satisfactory. A number of them have even been obtained on the operating table with a simple portable apparatus (the Siemens Sphere), placed at one metre and the exposure time being 8 to 12 seconds. It is obvious that more powerful machines should be used for preference, but it is useful to know that smaller ones can be used if necessary.

For the pelvis, a single plate is generally sufficient (but sometimes it can be useful to obtain two pictures, placed side by side) and then the Potter-Bucky diaphragm is used.

b) *Serial phlebography and two-exposure phlebography* - Arteriography has already demonstrated the need to obtain two successive radiograms of the same region with an interval of a few seconds between them, for the second film can reveal details of the arteriolar circulation which are invisible on the first. For this, two 30 x 40 cm frames which can be changed beneath the Potter-Bucky diaphragm are used.

In phlebography, successive exposures are even more important, for the customary slowness of the peripheral venous circulation and the low blood pressure levels mean that any obstacle to the flow of blood in a large vein is liable to cause a considerable slowing upstream, of the flow. Changes in the rate of flow are much more marked when the veins are damaged than when it is the arteries which are affected. This slowness of the venous blood flow is exaggerated even more in phlebography by the gap existing between the rate of flow of the venous blood and that of the contrast solutions used. I shall refer to this again.

The result of all this is that whereas the difference between exposure times in arteriography is a few seconds, in phlebography of the extremities, it is measured in tens of seconds. For the pelvis, where the venous blood flow is quicker, the differences are less.

In cases of venous disease, the additional phlebograms have nearly always provided details which are useful, and sometimes indispensable, in making a diagnosis.

Present experience seems to indicate that these exposures should be made at the 20th and 40th seconds after the first radiogram for the lower limbs, and it is sufficient to carry out these additional examinations on the thigh only, as the leg is always completely visualised in the first radiogram, which will therefore be the only one to cover the whole limb. The time elapsing between each exposure is sufficient for an assistant to be able to change the frame.

For the pelvis and upper limb, a single plate is generally used for the first phlebogram and one additional exposure is sufficient.

A table with a double base, enabling the frames to be put where desired, greatly facilitates successive changes. For the pelvis and upper limb, which require only a single film at a time and a single additional exposure, equipment designed for stereo-radiography, should be used.

Such are the indications at the present time as regards radiological technique, but they are not final and at the moment I am trying out a number of modifications which could have advantages.

The slow rate of progression of the contrast substance made me consider dividing the total radiography of a limb into two successive exposures, the leg to be radiographed first, and then the thigh. This would make it possible to reduce the amount injected by half and to carry out several examinations at the same session, if necessary. The results of a few trials were good for the leg but inadequate for the thigh, as interruption of the injection after the first radiogram (leg) diminishes the rate of progression of the contrast substance, which then only passes into the thigh very slowly and therefore undergoes greater dilution. To maintain the rate of flow of the solution in the veins, I then followed the injection with another of physiological saline at the same rate until the second exposure (thigh) had been made. The two successive radiograms of the thigh were then obtained in the usual way. I believe I can forecast that this technique will be a good one, but this remains to be proved.

c) *Stereo-phlebography and phleboscopy* - these are two procedures whose value will be obvious to everyone. The results already obtained by other workers, notably the British and Americans, have confirmed this but I have not yet tried them.

In short, the importance of phlebography seems to have been confirmed in:

the early diagnosis and location of the thrombus in acute phlebitis

the study of bypass venous networks in long-standing phlebitis, their topography and the disturbances following from them;

obtaining knowledge of what can be ascribed to anatomical lesions and to functional disturbances in the study of symptoms presented by various pathological conditions;

the differential diagnosis of oedema of the extremities, and in the diagnosis of acute venous thrombosis simulating arterial embolism;

investigations on the origin of varices and study of various aspects of this condition;

demonstration of the existence of venous spasm;

study of congenital venous disorders;

therapeutic outcome in venous disease.

CONCLUSIONS

It is quite difficult to set down in order, a plethora of assorted observations in a field where the technique has been constantly changing.

I have not always carried out the investigations that I should have done and I have sometimes introduced sudden modifications in the technique decided the evening before, after reflecting upon it.

Some cases could not be followed up and others did not have the additional examinations which would have supplied valuable information.

It is only when the whole is gathered together that the large gaps are perceived. This is necessary evil, but I hope that, in spite of everything, I have demonstrated the possibilities of the method, its essential principles, and some of the findings already made.

But it is one thing to understand the importance of a method and another to predict the future from it.

Any method of studying symptoms is characterised by two aspects. In the first place, it enables problems to be studied from a new point of view and brings to light facts which had remained unelucidated. Once such knowledge has been obtained, new examinations may not be necessary. The usefulness of the method consists precisely in providing a new basis for the development of new concepts of whatever kind. This value, however ephemeral it may be, is no less important because of the consequences which may result. It is the indication of what exists and does not change in each situation where the clinical picture is well established. But, on the other hand, it can provide information on conditions in which the external or other signs are incapable of doing so.

In such cases, the method should be used every time and should thus become a routine means of examination. For this it should be without danger and easy to carry out.

Phlebography is harmless and painless and the provisional technique has been laid down. I do not think that the fact that it requires four persons to carry it out is anything extraordinary, for the whole procedure cannot be reduced to the simplicity of a subcutaneous injection.

The final and the more transitory indications for phlebography can obviously be stated only after several years' work. There is an enormous amount to do. Not only do the possibilities which have already been recognised necessitate a large number of investigations, but there are also studies on new fields and new conditions to be considered. Pathological conditions affecting the mediastinum might benefit from being studied from the point of view of effects on the vessels which open into the superior vena cava. The territory of the portal vein is also quite a fascinating one.

One day, during a Talma operation, I injected a few cc of dilute Per-Abrodil into an omental vein and the very poor radiogram obtained gave me a very slight indication of the venous network of the liver. However, that did not lead any further at the time and it is experimental studies based on phlebography of the portal vein area which seem to me to have a future.

From the point of view of its immediate use in man, however, it is for the field of phlebography to be studied more thoroughly in relation to symptoms involving the extremities, where the various techniques can be put to the test either alternatively or simultaneously.

I would not like to finish without emphasising once again the importance of the therapeutic outcome demonstrated by phlebographic examinations. Thanks to them, early phlebitis, which once would not have been subjected to surgery, will probably gain from undergoing an emergency operation, whereas varices, whose treatment by surgery is still a matter of discussion, will be directly, with advantage, solely to methods of a medical nature, whether sclerosing or other, based on the principle of retrograde injection in association with stasis.

In short, I believe that the findings already obtained with phlebography have justified this presentation, and this is the only way that its real value can be determined.

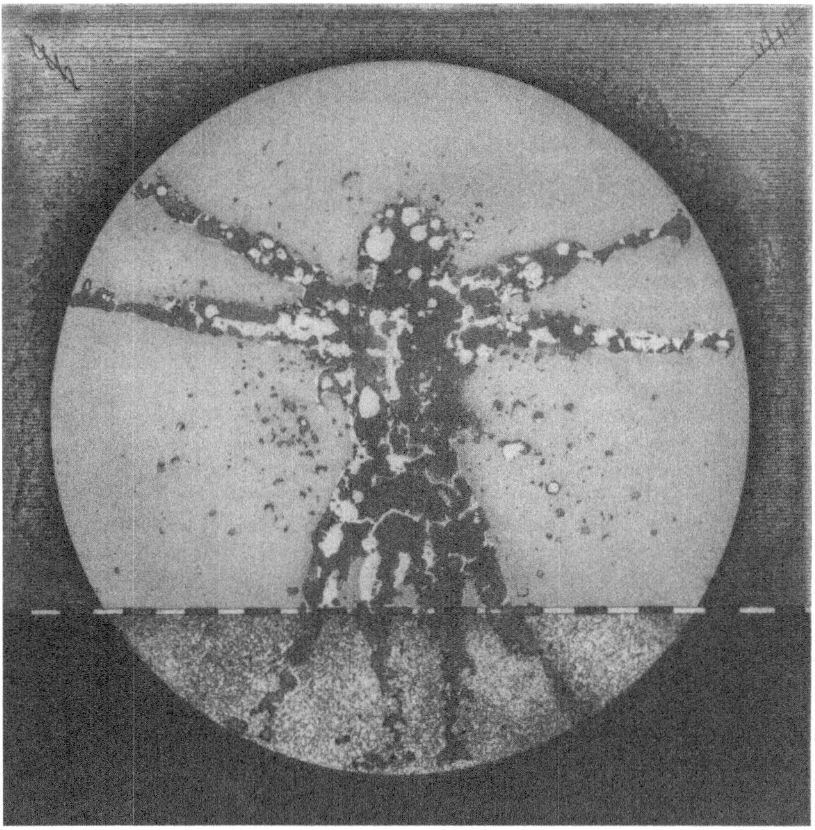

The dimension of man (1981) by Bartholomeu dos Santos, son of J. Cid dos Santos.

FIRST COMMUNICATION ON PORTOGRAPHY

A. de Sousa Pereira

(The method of phlebography in the study of disturbances of the portal circulation).
Lyon Chirurgical, 4, 6, 1951.

The difficulties encountered in the physio-pathological and surgical interpretation of some clinical syndromes in patients with disturbances involving the portal circulation led us to study the radiological visualisation of the portal system.

It is known that the portal system consists of veins coming from the abdominal part of the gastro-intestinal tract, the gall-bladder, the spleen and the pancreas and, meeting in a single trunk, form the origin of the portal vein, which, after bifurcations, divides into branches and terminates in the liver in the form of sinusoid capillaries.

However, quite considerable variations are observed in the morphology of the portal vein and its tributary branches, as has been shown recently by Douglass, Baggenstoss and Hollinshead. From a study of 92 human dissections, they reached the conclusion that the multiplicity of morphological variations makes it essential to identify the veins accurately before anastomoses are carried out on tributaries of the portal vein.

In the clinical interpretation of diseases presenting with signs of portal hypertension, it is particularly important to determine if the obstruction to the portal circulation is intra- or extra-hepatic. According to the site of the vascular obstruction, the portal hypertension is generalised or localised, and the surgical indications can be different in the two cases. In cases of intrahepatic obstruction, the portal circulation can be considered as deriving from the portal trunk or its tributary branches, but in cases of extra-hepatic obstruction the veins which can be used for anastomosis are solely those situated upstream of the site of the stenosis. These facts demonstrate the value of having information on the morphology of the portal vein and its tributary branches in surgery of portal hypertension.

Methods for the radiological visualisation of the portal vein and its tributary branches.

Study of all the areas supplied by the tributaries of the portal vein has led us to appreciate the need to inject the contrast medium into different veins, depending on the tributary to be visualised.

The portal vein, which is formed by the union of the superior mesenteric vein and the splenic vein, also receives the inferior mesenteric vein, which terminates in the splenic vein, the superior mesenteric vein or the confluence of these two veins. In addition, the portal vein receives the pancreatico-duodenal and pyloric veins directly, and in some cases the coronary veins and the right gastro-epiploic vein.

For visualisation of each of the areas supplied by the portal system we injected the opaque substance (Nosydrast) into a small branch vein originating there.

We carried out our first trials on visualisation of the superior mesenteric vein during appendicectomies for chronic appendicitis. At first, our aim was to obtain information on the disturbances of the ileo-caecal venous circulation which might accompany the inflammatory process in the appendix. During these investigations we observed that the injection of 20 cc of Nosydrast into the appendicular vein or a slender caecal, ileal or ileo-caecal vein passed through the mesenteric vein from its origin, visualised the main trunk of that vein, and so visualised the portal vein itself and its intrahepatic ramifying branches.

As injection of the contrast medium into this venous area enabled all the territory of the superior mesenteric vein and portal vein to be visualised, we followed the same technique in patients with portal hypertension. The results obtained were found to determine whether the obstruction to the portal circulation was intra-hepatic or extra-hepatic.

To obtain radiographic pictures of the *superior mesenteric vein* and the *portal vein,* we injected 20 cc of Nosydrast into the appendicular vein or a small ileo-caecal vein, after exposure of the caecum under local, or sometimes, general anaesthesia, radiography being carried out at the end of the injection. With this method, we obtained pictures of the superior mesenteric vein, the portal vein and its intra-hepatic branches. In some of our patients, we visualised the superior mesenteric vein and the portal vein by giving the injection into a vein of the ileum. However, as a rule we used a small appendicular or ileo-caecal vein, which enabled us to obtain a picture of the mesenteric vein from its origin.

We often obtained a picture of the intra-hepatic territory of the right branch and the portal bifurcation. In some cases, the intra-hepatic ramifications of the left branch of the portal vein were visible, but not so clearly as those of the right branch.

We have also given a lumbar paravertebral injection of 400 to 500 cc of oxygen into retroperitoneal cellular tissue before the intravenous injection of the contrast substance, and this showed the contours of the liver more accurately in the individual cases and gave a better contrast of the veins injected with the opaque product. However, we do not yet know if distension of the retroperitoneal tissue with oxygen alters the physiological conditions of circulation in the portal sysem.

To visualise the *inferior mesenteric vein* and its branches from their origin, we injected 20 cc of Nosydrast into a small submucosal dilatation of a rectal vein in the area of the anus, and made the exposure at the end of the injection. In that way, we were able to obtain a picture of the inferior mesenteric vein and its branches from their origin in patients with haemorrhoids or having thrombophlebitis of the rectal veins.

It is also possible to visualise the *splenic vein* by injecting the contrast substance into a vein in the hilus of the spleen. This we tried to do by making a transparietal puncture of the spleen.

It is also possible to visualise the *splenic vein* by injecting the contrast substance into a vein in the hilus of the spleen. This we tried to do by making a transparietal puncture of the spleen.

We have tried to visualise the gastric venous system, either by injecting into a vein in the omentum majus or into a gastro-epiploic vein. In spite of the proximity of the portal trunk, we were unable to obtain radiographic pictures of the extra- and intra-hepatic portal system which were any clearer than those given by injection of Nosydrast into the branches of the superior mesenteric vein from their origin.

The value of phlebographic studies in disturbances of the portal circulatory system

From the various findings that we have made so far we consider that phlebography of the portal vein and its tributaries is of obvious value in studying disturbances of the portal circulation.

In 15 patients with *chronic appendicitis*, as already mentioned, we carried out a phlebographic study of the ileo-caecal veins, branches originating in the superior mesenteric vein, during surgical operation.

In four of these cases, there were no radiographic signs of disturbances of the circulation in the veins of the caecum or meso-appendix or other branches of the superior mesenteric vein.

In contrast, in eleven cases the radiographic examination

revealed disturbances of the venous circulation: signs of phlebitis and venous spasm and even more or less extensive thrombophlebitis of the veins of the caecum and meso-appendix.

Phlebography of the *inferior mesenteric vein* made it possible to demonstrate either abnormal dilatation of veins, indicating the existence of haemorrhoids, or signs of thrombophlebitis in the branches originating in the inferior mesenteric vein.

In the *portal hypertension syndrome,* phlebography of the portal system, after a study of the venous tension in that system, gives very important information on the topography and nature of the venous obstruction. This fact can be demonstrated by a study of the two cases in which there were clinical and manometric signs of hypertension in the portal system and in which phlebographic study of this system was carried out by injection of the contrast substance into a tributary of the superior mesenteric vein.

The phlebographic study in the first of these patients confirmed that the obstruction to the portal circulation was extra-hepatic. The superior mesenteric vein showed gross dilatation in its upper segment, and, between the branches originating in the superior mesenteric vein and the veins of the abdominal wall, there were anastomoses indicating the existence of a collateral circulation derived from the general circulation. The trunk of the portal vein showed, near its origin at the confluence of the superior mesenteric vein and the splenic vein, a marked decrease in calibre over a stretch of about 3 centimetres, increasing again up to the bifurcation of this vein at the hepatic portal.

The second patient with a portal hypertension syndrome was also subjected to a phlebographic study by injection of the opaque medium into an ileo-caecal vein. The radiographic picture of the portal system in this patient showed that there was no obstruction to the circulation in the extra-hepatic territory of the portal system. The superior mesenteric vein is completely unobstructed from its origin to its termination. The extra-hepatic segment of the portal vein is seen to be uniformly dilated, and the opaque substance, after filling the portal vein and its intra-hepatic branches, flows back towards the splenic vein, which is equally dilated and visible as far as its branches at the hilus of the spleen. The disturbance to the intra-hepatic circulation led in addition to the development of a collateral circulation between the tributaries of the portal vein and the veins of the abdominal wall, and in the thorax, in the region of the tenth rib and the tenth intercostal space, venous anastomoses could be seen which seemed to have set up a substitute circulation with the tenth right intercostal vein.

The recent investigations by Thomas and Essex have shown that the injection of various substances, parasite extracts and anaphylactic shock can give rise to spasm of the veins of the liver, which may be sufficiently severe to block the flow of blood, bring about congestion of the liver, and raise the pressure in the portal system.

To determine whether constriction of hepatic veins could be related to states of portal hypertension, in this patient we carried out a series of six physiological interruptions of the splanchnic nerves and the first lumbar ganglion, on the right and left alternately. Favourable effects were observed, in particular an increase in urinary output and a decrease in the ascites. These findings led us to carry out a splanchnicectomy and a lumbar sympathectomy (LI-LII) on the right side.

Phlebographic study of the portal system a fortnight later revealed new conditions in the portal circulatory system. An injection was given into a branch originating in the superior mesenteric vein at the same site and under similar conditions as for the pre-operative phlebography. However, the post-operative phlebographic study showed that there was no longer any stasis in the splenic vein, that the anastomoses between the veins of the liver and the right tenth intercostal vein were no longer visible, that the trunk of the portal vein was slightly smaller in calibre, and that the intra-hepatic ramifications of the portal vein were more clearly seen than before the operation. In the lumbar region anastomoses still persisted which seemed to connect the portal circulatory system with the veins of the posterior abdominal wall.

The findings in this patient suggest the possible existence of spasm of the intra-hepatic venous branches, a condition which seems to be susceptible to the favourable effect of functional or surgical interruption of the sympathetic innervation of the portal system.

CONCLUSION

The results of investigations on phlebography of the portal system demonstrate the practical possibility of visualising this system by radiography after the injection of an opacifying substance into a tributary of the portal vein.

Depending on the territory of the tributaries of the portal vein to be visualised, the injection is given into the territory of the superior mesenteric vein, the inferior mesenteric vein, the splenic vein, or the gastro-epiploic or gastric veins.

Phlebography of the tributaries of the portal system makes it possible to demonstrate pathological disturbances in the areas supplied by these veins, such as thromboses, spasm, and dilatations. In cases of portal hypertension, this method can provide information on the extra-hepatic or intra-hepatic topography and the nature of the obstruction to the portal circulation.

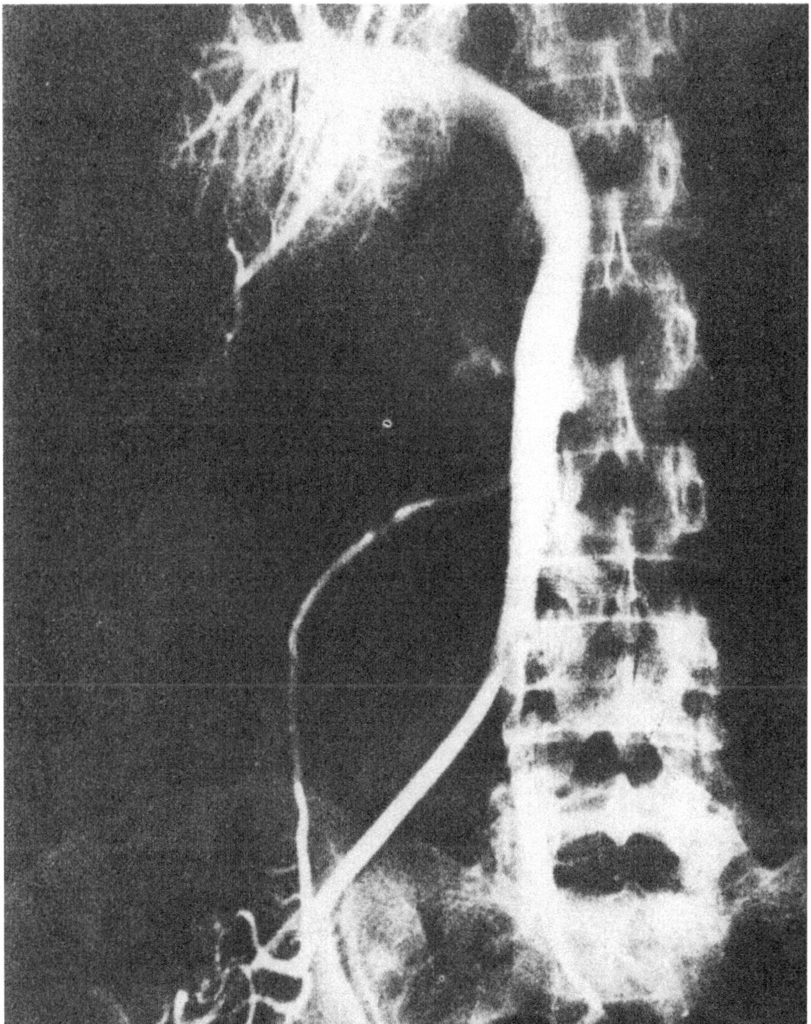

Portography A. de Sousa Pereira

THE DEVELOPMENT OF IODINATED ORGANIC CONTRAST MEDIA

by Moses Swick

Modern radiology is indebted to the work of the Portuguese School but is also dependent upon the pioneers of other countries notably Germany and the United States of America. An outstanding figure with experience of both these countries is Moses Swick, Urologist of Mount Sinai Hospital, New York, for it was he who first used iodinated organic compounds in radiology and it is the development of these compounds which are in use today. What follows is a resumé of Swick's work provided by himself.

"At age 28 I was chosen from the interns at Mount Sinai Hospital to receive the Emanuel Libman Fellowship to continue my studies in Germany with particular reference to the field of Urology. One of the clinics at which I worked was the medical service of Prof. Leopold Lichtwitz at the Staedisches Krankenhaus Hamburg-Altona. It was here that my basic definitive work, leading to the successful discovery of Uroselectan (lopax in America) was initiated.

At that time, Prof. Lichtwitz was trying out a compound, Selectan Neutral, against infections in man (Selectan Neutral is an lodo pyridon N methyl compound) which had been synthesized by Prof. Artur Binz of the Agriculture College of Berlin and had been utilized in the cow against mastitis without much success.

At that time, I was not familiar with any work at visualizing the urinary system either by mouth or intravenously. The only knowledge that I possessed was that the lodine element possessed excellent roentgenologic opaque properties. The additional knowledge based on my premedical studies was that an element bound to an aromatic organic nucleus was tightly bound, not ionizable as in the inorganic sodium iodide. It occurred to me that Selectan Neutral might be valuable in visualizing the urinary system based on excretion studies. Prof. Lichtwitz was very kind in affording me the facilities to experiment with Selectan Neutral - a spot in the laboratory (Chemistry), animals (rabbits and dogs), the X-ray Department facilities, and its use in the animals; excretion studies (urine), simultaneous X-ray studies, and its application in man. Having established that the rabbit could tolerate 0.2 grams per kilogram of body weight, I administered the Selectan Neutral to the human. Excretion studies revealed that 75 to 80% of the injected iodine could be recovered in the urine. The results in man were encouraging but not ideal; the outline of the urinary bladder could be visualized radiologically, the renal pelvis at times very faintly, the renal parenchyma accentuated. There were side effects, but not so intolerable as to be discouraging. In one case, that of a high occluding ureteric stone, satisfactory visualization of the upper urinary tract was observed. Purely on an empirical basis, it occurred to me that the methyl radical might be an offending factor. Thus, the desired results might be obtained by a substitution of the methyl radical, an increase of the iodine content of the compound, and increase in the solubility.

With Prof. Lichtwitz's permission, I visited Prof. Binz in Berlin who was not aware of my investigations, at which time I submitted my observations. Accordingly he furnished me with a compound, - a double iodo N pyridon with the methyl radical substituted with an acetic acid radical - this was insoluble. Upon returning to Berlin again, another compound, a diiodo-N-pyridone acetic acid salt of sodium - somewhat more soluble but still not sufficiently so.

In order to be in close contact with Prof. Binz and with Prof. Lichtwitz's permission, I transferred my work to Berlin, utilizing the clinical material at the Urologic Service of Prof. von Lichtenberg at the St. Hedwigs Hospital. Prof. von Lichtenberg had no knowledge of the nature of the compound Selectan Neutral that I was investigating.

I continued with the intravenous application, observations and X-ray studies with Selectan Neutral in man awaiting modifications of the iodo-pyridone compound. Prof. von Lichtenberg was attending an American Urologic Association meeting in the States while I was continuing my studies. In his absence by a stroke of luck, Binz sent me samples of mono iodo-pyridone N acetate of sodium salt (Uro-Selectan). This synthesis had been accomplished by Binz in 1925 but had not previously been assessed for medical use.

Uroselectan met all my requirements. Rabbits could tolerate 3 grams per kilogram of body weight, was excreted in high concentration in the urine, 85-95% was excreted in the urine unchanged. There were no side effects. It was highly soluble (42%) and yielded excellent intravenous urinary roentgenograms - about 75% of the substance was recovered in the urine in the first two hours.

I telegraphed Dr. Libman of my success and to inform Prof. von Lichtenberg in the States of the gratifying results with Uroselectan. Upon the latter's return to St. Hedwigs, I was informed that he considered presenting the paper together with me at the 9th Kongress of the German Urologic Association meeting in Munich in September of 1929. I objected, so did Prof. Lichtwitz in Hamburg. Lichtwitz informed Dr. Salle - editor of the Klinische Wochenschrift. At a meeting of all parties, it was agreed that I would present my paper followed by a second paper by Von Lichtenberg and Swick on the Klinische Prufung which were published as such in the November issue of 1929.

After the 9th Kongress, we visited Milano and Genoa with the same unfortunate experiences. At this point I decided to return to New York - December 1929.

At Mount Sinai Hospital, I continued my work with Uroselectan, both clinically and in the laboratory.

In the course of my work at Mount Sinai, I came upon the idea that the iodide element could be organically bound to an aromatic nucleus, representing a product of metabolism - that was Hippuric acid. It had been known that benzoic acid is detoxified in the liver by glycine to form hippuric acid (Hippus, the product of metabolism in the horse). Man excretes about 1 gram in 24 hours. Sodium benzoate is the preservative i.e. in catsup (Tomato Ketchup). The attempts at the synthesis of hippuran was initially carried out in the chemistry laboratory of Mount Sinai Hospital under the supervision of Dr. Harry Sabatka, but shortly thereafter discontinued. I then contacted Sachs with the Zenith Corporation where small amounts of the sodium salt of iodo-hippuric acid (Iodo-Hippuran) was synthesized and which I investigated in the laboratory in rabbits and in man.

After my initial success with Iodo-Hippuran, I turned the compound over to the Mallinckrodt Chemical Works where the chemist Dr. Wallingford collaborated with me in its production for commercial use. Iodo Hippuran is a mono iodo benzoic acid nucleus compound and is the forerunner and stimulus of our present compounds, diatrizoate (Hypaque Urografin), iothalamate (Conray) which are all salts of triiodic benzoic acids*"

Moses Swick

Urologist, New York, U.S.A. 1981

(Editorial Note:
*These latter compounds are salts of substituted of benzoic acids which are detoxified by 2 acetyl - amino groups at C3 + C5. Three atoms of iodine are placed at C2, C4, C6 positions to provide the necessary radio opacity).

BIBLIOGRAPHY

PIONEERS IN RADIOLOGY — EGAS MONIZ

1. L'encéphalographie artérielle, son importance dans la localisation des tumeurs cérébrales — *Revue Neurologique* — 1927 — 48: 72 — Separata de 18 pp.
2. Injections intracarotidiennes et substances injectables opaques aux rayons X — *Presse Médicale* — 1927 — no. 63 — Separata de 19 pp.
3. A prova da encefalografia arterial — *Lisboa Médica* — 1927 — 4: 301 — Separata de 50 pp.
4. La radioartériographie cérébrale — Académie de Médecine de Paris — Séance du 12 Juillet 1927 — *Bulletin de l'Académie de Médecine* — 1927 — XCVIII — Separata de 5 pp.
5. Radiografia das artérias cerebrais — *Journal da Sociedade das Ciências Médicas de Lisboa* — 1927 — 91 — Separata de 14 pp.
6. Considérations anatomiques sur le paquet sylvien vu à la radiographie chez le vivant — *Arquivo de Anatomia e Antropologia* — 1928 — 11: 301 — Separata de 13 pp.
7. A encefalografia arterial no diagnóstico dos tumores cerebrais — (Conferência realizada na Academia de Medicina do Rio de Janeiro). *Boletim da Academia Nacional de Medicina* — 1928 — 19: 321.
8. L'encéphalographie artérielle — *Journal de Médecine de Bordeaux* — 1928 no. 23: 915.
9. L'encéphalographie artérielle et le diagnostic d'une tumeur de la partie antérieure du lobe temporal gauche — Em colaboração com Almeida Lima — *Encéphale* — 1928 — 15: 196 — Separata de 4 pp.
10. L'épreuve de l'encéphalographie artérielle dans le diagnostic de quatre cas de tumeurs cérébrales opérés — Em colaboração com Almeida Lima e Amândio Pinto — Separata de 31 pp.
11. A estereoscopia de encefalografia arterial no vivo (Primeiras provas obtidas) — Communicação feita ă Academia das Ciências de Lisboa — Sessão de 11 de Março de 1928.

12. Localisation d'une tumeur du lobe temporal par l'encéphalographie artérielle.— Comunicação à Academia das Ciências de Lisboa — 1928.
13. Les méthodes radiodiaphoriques dans la localisation des tumeurs cérébrales. Nouvelle technique radiologique de l'encéphalographie artérielle — *Revue Neurologique* — 1928 — 2: 20 — Separata de 5 pp.
14. Un nouveau cas de diagnostic de tumeur cérébrale *post mortem* par l'encéphalographie artérielle — Em colaboração com Almeida Lima - *Revue Neurologique* — 1928 — 2: 27.
15. Nouvelle technique de l'encéphalographie artérielle. Quelques cas de localisation de tumeurs cérebrales — *Presse Médicale* — 1928 — no. 44.
16. La radioartériographie et la topographie cranio-encéphalique — Em colaboração com Almeida Lima e Almeida Dias — *Jornal de Radiologie et d'Électrologie* — 1928 — 12: 72.
17. A técnica da encefalografia arterial no homem; sua importância na localização das neoplasias cerebrais — Actas do III Congresso Nacional de Medicina — 1928 — 1: 123.
18. Tumeur cérébrale localisée par l'encéphalographie artérielle. Opération — *Revue Neurologique* — 1928 — 2: 237.
19. Die arterielle Encephalographie als Methode zur lokâlisierung von Hirntumoren — *Klinische Wochenschrift* — 1929 — 8: 118.
20. A encefalografia arterial como subsidio operatório — *A Medicina Contemporânea* — 1929 — 47: 270.
21. A arteriografia cerebral na meningite serosa circunscrita — Comunicação à Academia das Ciências de Lisboa — *A Medicina Contemporânea* — 1929 — 47: 96.
22. L'artériographie cérébrale par l'épreuve de l'encéphalographie artérielle — Em colaboração com Amândio Pinto e Almeida Lima.
24. Diagnóstico encefalográfico dos tumores cerebrais — Comunicação à Corporação dos Assistentes do Hospital Escolar de Lisboa — *A Medicina Contemporânea* — 1929 — no. 17.
25. Encefalografia arterial. A propósito de las injecciones carotídeas — *Revista Oto-Neuro-Oftalmológica y de Cirugia Neurológica de Buenos Aires* — 1929 —4: 276.
26. L'encéphalographie artérielle — *Bruxelas-Médical* — 1929 — no. 19: 547.
27. L'épreuve encéphalographie dans un cas de tumeurs multiples du cerveau — Em colaboração com Almeida Line — *Revue*

Neurologique — 1929 — 1: 1142 13: 429 — *Comptes-rendus Société de Biologie* — 1929 — 101: 981.
28. Sobre a circulação dos meningiomas —*Portugal Medico— 1929* —13: 429
29. Le syndrome de la pseudohypertension crânienne artérioscléreuse. Aspects radioartériographiques — *Encéphale* — 1929 — 16: 337.
30. Aspectos arteriográficos del cérebro en los casos de tumor del lobulo frontal — Em colaboração com Amândio Pinto e Almeida Lima — *Revista Médica de Barcelona* — 1930 — 14: 38 — Separata de 10 pp.
31. Aspectos arteriográficos num caso de tumor da giândula pineal e tubérculos quadrigémios — *Lisboa Médica* — 1930 — 7: 368.
32. Aspects artériographiques du cerveau dans les tumeurs de la fosse cérébelleuse — Em colaboração com Almeida Lima — *Revue Neurologique* — 1930 — 1:54 — Separata de 9 pp.
33. Le diagnostic des tumeurs cérébrales par l'encéphalographie artérielle — *Clinique et Laboratoire* — 1930 — no. 5, 97.
34. Tumeur de la glande pinéale, irriguée par un seul des groupes sylviens. Diagnostic par l'épreuve encéphalographique — Em colaboração com Amândio Pinto e Almeida Lima — *Revue Neurologique* — 1930 1: 51 — Separata de 4 pp.
35. Alguns casos de tumores cerebrais tornados visiveis pela prova encefalográfica — Em colaboração com Amândio Pinto e Almeida Lima — *Revista Oto-Neuro-Oftalmológica y de Cirugia Neurolgica* — 1931 — 6: 316.
36. Alguns novos aspectos das encefalografias arteriais — (Comunicação feita à Sociedade das Ciências Médicas em 10 de Dezembro de 1931) — *A Medicina Contemporânea* — 1931.
37. Angiopneumographie — Em colaboração com Lopo de Carvalho e Almeida Lima — *Presse Médicale* — 1931 — no. 53 — Separata de 23 pp.
38. Arterial encephalography and its value in the diagnosis of brain tumors — Em colaboração com Amândio Pinto e Almeida Lima — *Surgery, Gynaecology and Obstetrics* — 1931 — 56: 155 — Separata de 14 pp.
39. Aus dem Gebiete der Angiopneumographie. Vorläufige Mitteilung — Em colaboração com Lopo de Carvalho e Almeida Lima — *Beiträge zur Klinik der Tuberkulose* — 1931 — 79: 72.

40. La circulation veineuse du cou et la décharge veineuse de l'encéphale — Em colaboração com Lopo de Carvalho e Almeida Lima — *Comptes rendus des séances de la Société de Biologie, section Portugaise* — 1931 — 107: 84.

41. Diagnostic des tumeurs cérébrales et épreuve de l'encéphalographie artérielle (Préface de Monsieur le Docteur J. Babinski) — Paris. *Masson* — 1931 Volume de 511 pp. e 225 figs. originais.

42. Diagnostic encéphalographique des tumeurs cérébrales par visibilité et déplacement des artéres — Em colaboração com Amândio Pinto e Almeida Lima — *Bordeaux Chirurgical* — 1931 — 2: 7.

43. La encefalografia arterial — (Conferência realizada em Saragoça a pedido da Associação Neuropsiquiátrica Espanhola, em Septembro de 1930) — *Arquivos de Neurobiologia* — 1931 —11: 504.

44. La localisation des tumeurs cérébrales par l'encéphalographie artérielle — (Rapport présenté au Congrés Neurologique Internacional de Berne) — *Revue Neurologique* — 1931 — 2: 371 — *Lisboa Médica* — 1931 — 8: 559 — *Revista Oto-Neuro-Oftalmológica y de Cirurgia Neurlógica* — 1931 — 6: 455.

45. A propos de l'article "Nouvelle méthode de radiographie des artères et des veines sur le vivant, ses applications cliniques au diagnostic" — *Presse Médicale* — 1931 — No. 4 — Separata de 3 pp.

46. A prova encefalográficia por injecções livres na carótid interna e na carótida primitiva — Em colaboração com Almeida Lima — *A Medicina Contemporânea* — 1931 — 49: 229 — *Jornal da Sociedade de Ciéncias Médicas de Lisboa* — 1931 — 95: 187.

47. Reflexões a propósito de dois casos de tumores do lobo frontal com prova encefalográfica — *Acta Médica Latina* — 1931 — 20: 103.

48. Resultados do emprego do "thorotrast" na prova da encefalografia arterial — (Comunicação feita à Academia das Ciências de Lisboa em 29 de Outubro de 1931) — Em colaboração com Amândio Pinto e Almeida Lima — *A Medicina Contemporânea* — 1931 — 49: 399 — Separata de 11 pp.

49. Le thorotrast dans l'encéphalographie artérielle — Em colaboração com Amândio Pinto e Almeida Lima — (Comunicação à Société de Neurologie de Paris em 5 de Novembro de 1931) — *Revue Neurologique* — 1931 — 38: 646.

50. Tumeurs cérébrales visibles par l'épreuve encéphalographique — Em colaboração com Amândio Pinto e Almeida Lima — *Lyon Chirurgical* — 18: 273 — Separata de 9 pp.
51. Tumores cerebrais tornados visiveis pela encefalografia — Trabalho apresentado ao. Colégio de Cirurgiões pelo Prof. A. Brandão (filho) — 1931.
52. A visibilidade aos raios X dos vasos pulmonares obtida por injecções de liquido opaco na auricula direita — Em colaboracão com Lopo de Carvalho e Almeida Lima — (Comunicação à Academia das Ciências de Lisboa em 19 de Fevereiro de 1931) — *Boletim da Academia das Cieñcias de Lisboa* — 1931 — 3: 145 — *Bulletin de l'Académie de Médecine de Paris* — 1931 — 105: 627.
53. A visibilidade dos vasos pulmonares. Primeiros ensaios de angiopneumografia — (Comunicação á Sociedade dê Ciências Médicas de Lisboa em Março de 1931) — Em colaboração com Lopo de Carvalho e Almeida Lima — *A Medicina Contemporânea* — 1931 40: 95.
54. Alguns aspectos da encefalografia arterial — *A Medicina Contemporânea* 1932 — no. 1 — p. 23.
55. L'angiopneumographie et son aplication dans la tuberculose pulmonaire -- Em colaboração com Lopo de Carvalho e Almeida Lima — *Presse Médicale* — 1932 — 40: 1098 — Separata de 16 pp.
56. L'artério-phlébographie comme moyen de déterminer la vitesse de la circulation du cerveau, des méninges et des parties molles du crâne — *Bulletin de l'Académie de Médecine* — 1932 — 107: — 316 — Separata de 3 pp. — *Annales de Médecine* — 1932 — 32: 193 — Separata de 28 pp.
57. Aspectos radiográficos da cirulação cerebral. Sua importância clinica — *Revista de Radiologia Clinica* — 1932 — 1: 393 — Separata de 11 pp.
58. L'aspect à l'épreuve encéphalographique des angiomes artérielles dans le domaine de la carotid interne — Em colaboração com Cancela de Abreu e Cándido de Oliveira — *Revue Neurologique* — 1932 — 2: 165.
59. Aspects anatomiques, physiologiques et cliniques de l'artériographie cérébrale. Nouvelle technique par le thorotrast — *Revue Médicale de la Suisse Romande* — 1932 — 32: 193.
60. Nuevos aspectos de la angiografia cerebral — *Revista Oto-Neuro-Oftalmológica y de Cirugia Neurológica Sud-Americana* — 1932 — 7: 1012 — Separata de 39 pp.

61. Paraplégie et macrogénitosomie précoce dans un cas d'hydrocéphalie congénitale avec os du crâne épais. Aspects en "pattes d'araignée"de la circulation cérébrale des hydrocéphaliques — Em colaboração com Almeida Lima — *Revue Neurologique* — 1932 — 1: 693.

62. Phlébographie cérébrale. Essais de détermination de la vitesse du sang dans les cappilaires du cerveau chez l'homme — Em colaboração com Almeida Lima — *Comptes-rendus des séances de la Société de Biologie, secion portugaise* — 1932 — 109: 1037.

63. Los progresos de la angiografia — *Revista Médica de Barcelona* — 1932 — 18: 462 — Separata de 10 pp.

64. Os seios venosos da dura mater, sua visibilidade aox raios X — Em colaboração com Abel Alves e Fernando de Almeida — *Lisboa Médica* — 1932 — 9: 523 — Separata de 16 pp.

65. Sintomatologia neurológica e arteriográfica dum volumoso tumor do lobo frontal esquerdo — *Hygia* — 1932 — 1: 3.

66. Sur la capacité des capillaires cérébraux — *Comptes-rendus des séances de la Société de Biologie, section portugaise* — 1932 — 110: 1034.

67. Vantagens do método arterioflebográfico no estudo da velocidade de circulação do sangue no homem — (Comunicação feita à Sociedade de Ciências Médicas de Lisboa em 27 de Fevereiro de 1932 — *A Medicina Contemporânea* —1932 — no. 10 — Separata de 9 pp.

68. Visibilidades aos raios X das veias profundas do cérebro — Em colaboração com Fernando de Almeida e Abel Alves — *Lisboa Médica* — 1932 — 9: 587 — Separata de 12 pp.

69. A visibilidade dos vasos pulmonares (angiopneumografia) — Em colaboração com Lopo de Carvalho, Aleu Saldanha, Almeida Lima, José Rocheta, V. Lacerda, A. Carvalho e C. Vidal — *Lisboa Médica* — 1932 — 9: 431 — Separata de 34 pp.

70. Visibilidade das veias do cérebro pela prova encefalográfica — Flebografia normal — Em colaboração com Almeida Lima — *Lisboa Médica* — 1932 — 9: 201.

71. La visibilité des sinus de la dure-mére par l'épreuve encéphalographique — Em colaboração com Abel Alves e Fernando de Almeida – *Presse Médicale*— 1932 — 40: 1499 — Separata de 20 pp.

72. La visibilité des vaisseaux pulmonaires (angiopneumographie) — Em colaboração com Lopo de Carvalho e Aleu Saldanha — *Journal de Radiologie et d'Electrologie* — 1932 16: 469 — Separata de 13 pp.

73. Die Vorzüge des Thorotrast bei arterieller Enzephalographie — Em colaboração com Amândio Pinto e Almeida Lima — *Röntgenpraxis* — 1932 — 4: 90 — Separata de 4 pp.

74. Anévrisme intracranien de la carotide interne droite rendu visible par l'angiographie cérébrale — *Revue d'Oto-Neuro-Ophtalmolgie* — 1933 — 11: 746 — Publicado em espanhol na *Revista Oto-Neuro-Oftalmológica y de Cirugia Neurlógica Sud Americana* — 1934 — 9: 225.

75. L'angiografia cerebrale — Archivio de Radiologia — 1933 no 4 — Separata de 16 pp.

76. L'angiographie cérébrale chez le vivant, son importance anatomique — *Folio Anatomica Universitatis Conimbrigensis* — 1933 — 8: 1.

77. Artériographie du cervelet et des autres organes de la fosse postérieure — Em colaboração com Amândio Pinto e Abel Alves — *Bulletin de l'Académie de Médicine de Paris* — 1933 — 109.

78. Aspecto flebográfico de um meningioma — Em colaboração com Almeida Lima — (Comunicação à Academia das Ciências de Lisboa em 16 de Dezembro de 1932) — *A Medicina Contemporânea* — 1933 — 31: 6.

79. Cerebral angiography, its application in clinical practice and physiology — *Lancet* — 1933 — 2: 1144.

80. Cerebral angiography with thorotrast — *Archives of Neurology and Psychiatry* — 1933 — 29: 1318.

81. Circulation artérielle capillaire et veineuse des méningiomes — Em colaboração com Almeida Lima — *Vol. Jubilaire de Marinesco* — 1933 — p. 467 — *Anales de Medicina* — 1933 — 32 — Separata de 8 pp.

82. Consideraciones sobre la angiografia normal y patológica del cerebro — *Acta Ciba* — 1933 — no. 7, p. 157.

83. A filmagem da circulação cerebral — Em colaboração com Almeida Lima e Pereira Caldas — *A Medicina Contemporânea* — 1933 — 51: 19 — Separata de 7 pp.

84. L'importance diagnostique de l'artériographie de la fosse postérieure — Em colaboração com Abel Alves — *Revue Neurologique* — 1933 — 2: 91 — Separata de 6 pp.

85. Interpretação das opacidades nas séries angiográficas da cabeça —Em colaboração com Abel Alves e Pereira Caldas — *Lisboa Médica* — 1933 — 10: 122. — Separata de 26 pp.

86. A prova encefalográfica do cérebro feita dos dois lados na mesma sessão operatória — Em colaboração com Abel Alves — *Revista de Radiologia Clinica* — 193 — no 2 — Separata de 2 pp — *Revue Neurologique* — 1933 — 1: 375 — Separata de 2 pp.

87. A prova angiográfica nos casos de aneurismas e angiomas cerebrais (Comunicação à Academia das Ciências de Lisboa em 22 de Dezembro e 1933 — *Boletim da Academia das Ciências de Lisboa* — 1933 — 6: 485.
88. Le sinus droit et l'ampoule de Gallen opacifiés par la voie du tronc basilaire — Em colaboração com Fernando de Almeida — *Lisboa Médica* — 1933 — 10: 587 — Separata de 11 pp.
89. Tronc basilaire et artères dérivées — *Encéphale* — 1933 — 28: 705.
90. Troubles circulatoires du cerveau produits par des tumeurs cérébrales dans le voisinage du syphon carotidien — Em colaboração com Almeida Lima e Diogo Furtado — *Presse Médicale* — 1933 — no 55 — Separata de 16 pp.
91. - Visibilidade aos raios X do tronco basilar, aretéria cerebal posterior e artérias cerebelosas — (Comunicação Sociedade das Ciências Médicas de Lisboa em 1 de Junho de 1933) — Em colaboração com Amândio Pinto e Abel Alves — *A Medicina Contemporânea* 1933 — 51: 141 — Separata de 7 pp.
92. Visibilidade em série da circulação cerebral tornada visivel pelo iodeto de sódio e pelo thorotrast — Em colaboração com Abel Alves, Pereira Caldas e Diogo Furtado — *Lisboa Médica* — 1933 — 10: 111 — Separatade 15 pp.
93. Visibilité aux rayons X des veines temporales superficielles et occipitales — Em colaboração com Diogo Furtado — *Folia Anatomica Universitatis Conimbrigenis* — 1933 — 8: 1 — Separata de 2 pp.
94. The visibility of the pulmonary vessels (Angiopneumography) — Em colaboração com Lopo de Carvalho — *Acta Radiológica* — 1933 — 14: 433.
95. L'angiographie cérébrale. Ses applications et résultats en anatomie, physiologie et clinique — Paris. *Masson* — 1934 — Um volume de 327 pp. ilustrado com 192 figuras originais.
96. Angiographies en série de la circulation de la tête — Em colaboração com Almeida Lima e Pereira Caldas — *Revue Neurologique* — 1934 — 1: 489 — Separata de 22 pp.
97. La barrera capilar en el cerebro y en los tejidos de la cabeza — *Boletin de la Universidade de Santiago de Compostela* — 1934 — Número especial *in memoriam* do Prof. Cadarso — Separata de 7 pp.
98. L'épreuve angiographique dans les cas d'abcès cérébraux — Em colaboração com Romão Loff — *Bordeaux Chirurgical* — 1934 — 5: 1.

99. L'evolution de la technique de l'angiographie cérébrale — *Progrés Médical* — 1934 — no. 46 — Separata de 8 pp.

100. Les hématomes sous-arachnoidiens et les anévrismes cérébraux — *Presse Médicale* — 1934 — noo 50 — Separata de 20 pp.

101. La phlébographie dans l'hémorragie cérébrale profonde — *Revue Neurologique* — 1934 — 2: 886.

102 A visibilidade das veias profundas do cérebro, importância de sua deformação e deslocação como elemento de diagnóstico em alguns casos de tumores cerebrais — (Comunicação à Academia das Ciências de Lisboa em 7 de Junho de 1934) — *Boletim da Academia das Ciências de Lisboa* — 1934 — 52: 199.

103. Angiomes cérébraux. Importance de l'angiographie cérébrale dans leur diagnostic — *Bulletin de l'Académie de Médecine* — 1935 — 13: 174 — *Presse Médicale* — 1935 — No. 13, p. 246 — Separata de 10pp.

104. A angiografia no diagnóstic dos aneurismas e angiomas do cérebro — *Lisboa Médica* — 1935 — 12: 455 — Separata de 12 pp. — *Comptes-rendus of the Internacional Congress of Neurology, London* — 1935 — *Revue Neurologique* — 1935 —2: 625.

105. Tumores da fossa posterior. Aspectos arteriográficos do cérebro nas dilatações ventriculares — *A Medicina Contemporânea* — 1935 — no 11 — Separata de 15 pp.

106. Aspectos arteriográficos e flebográficos dos meningiomas da asa do esfenóide — *Lisboa Médica* — 1935 12: 399 — Separata de 13 pp.

107. Aumento de circulação do diplóico da calote craniana na doença óssea de Paget — Em colaboração com Almeida Dias e Luis Pacheco — *Lisboa Médica* — 1935 — 12: 114 — Separata de 15 pp.

108. Avantages de l'épreuve angiographique dans la carotide primitive — *Clinica, Higiene e Hidrologia* — 1935 — no 9: 343 — Separata de 3 pp.

109. Résultats cliniques et physiologiques de l'angiographie cérébrale — (Conferência feita na Semaine Médicale Internationale en Suisse, Montreux — *Schweitzerische Medizinische Wochenschrift* — 1935 — no. 47 — Separata de 14 pp.

110. A angiografia cerebral no diagnóstico das lesões vasculares do cérebro — (Comunicação à Academia das Ciências de Lisboa em 2 de Julho de 1936) — *Boletim da Academia das Ciências de Lisboa* — 1936 — 8: 222 — *Minerva Médica* — 1943.
111. A angiografia cerebral ao serviço da clinica — *Coimbra Médica* — 1936 — 3: 317.
112. Obstrução da carótida interna à altura da carótida primitiva, denuniciada pela arteriografia — (Comunicação à Academia das Ciências de Lisboa em 9 de Janeiro de 1936) — Em colaboração com Almeida Lima e Ruy de Lacerda — *Boletim da Academia das Ciências de Lisboa* — 1936 — 8: 17 — *A Medicina Contemporánea* — 1936 — 54: 118.
113. Radiodiagnostic de la circulation cérébrale (Angiographie cérébraie) — Rapport présenté à la Réunion Neurologique Internationale de Paris, 26 e 27 de Maio de 1936 *Revue Neurologique* — 1936 1: 1359 — Separata de 30 pp.
114. Arteriografia acidental da fossa posterior por injecção na artéria vertebral — (Comunicação à Academia das Ciências de Lisboa em 3 de Junho de 1937) — Em colaboração com Joaquim Imaginário — *Boletim da Academia das Ciências de Lisboa* — 1937 — 9: 225.
115. Déformations des sinus droit et longitudinal inférieur et des veines profondes du cereveau dans le diagnostic des néoplasies cérébales — *Zentralblatt für Neurochirurgie* — 1937 — 2: 213 — Separata de 12 pp.
116. Idees générales sur l'angiographie cérébrale — *Bolletino dell'Associazione Médica Triestina* — 1937 — 15 — Separata de 17 pp.
117. A propos de l'artériographie de la fosse postérieure. Anomalie de position de l'artère verteAbrale occupant la place de la carotide interne— Em colaboração com Joaquim Imaginário — *A Medicina Contemporânea* — 1937 — no 22 — Separata de 12 pp.
118. Visibilité de la jugulaire interne chez le vivant — *Folia Anatomica Universitatis Conimbrigensis* — 1937 — 12 — Separata de 5 pp.
119. Alterações do calibre da comunicante anterior em casos de lesões vasculares do cérebro — (Comunicação à Academia das Ciências de Lisboa em 2 de Junho de 1938) — *Boletim da Academia das Ciências de Lisboa* — 1938 — 10: 121.
120. Circulation double d'un angiome cérébrale — *Zentralblatt fur Neurochirurgie* — 1938 — 3: 217.
121. Clinica della angiografia cerebraie — Torino, I.T.E.R., — 1938 — Volume de 142 pp. e 42 figuras.

122. L'hyperostose frontale interne. Étude angiographique d'un cas chez une jeune femme. Syndrome de Morgagni — Stewart — Morel — Schizofrenie — 1938 — 7: 223 — Separata de 18 pp.
123. As más arteriografias cerebrais podem induzir em erros de diagnóstico — *Actas Ciba* — 1938 — 5.
124. Visibilité par contraste des gaines vasculo-nerveuses du cou et leurs prolongements — Em colaboração com Luis Pacheco e Joaquim Imaginário — *Imprensa Médica* — 1938 — no 18: 295 — Separata de 18 pp.
125. Alterações angiográficas nos tumores da porção anterior do corpo caloso — Em colaboração com Almeida Lima — *Imprensa Médica* — 1940 — no 11.
126. Die cerebrale Arteriographie und Phlebographie — Berlin, Springer — 1940 — Um volume de VIII-413pp., illustrado com 324 figuras.
127. Diagnóstico radiológico das obstruções carotideas — *Boletim da Sociedade Portuguesa de Radiologia Médica* — 1940 — no 1.
128. A fotografia da circulação normal e patológica do cérebro — (Comunicação à Academia das Ciências de Lisboa em 7 de Março de 1940).
129. Angiomas profundos do cérebro — Em colaboração com Almeida Lima — *Lisboa Médica* — 1941 —18: 213 — Separata de 10 pp.
130. Trombosis y otras obstrucciones de las carótidas — Barcelona, *Salvat* — 1941 — Um volume de 173 pp., illustrado com 67 figuras.
131. Tumores da glândula pineal. Diagnóstico angiográfico — *Actas Españolas de Neurologia y Psiquiatria* — 1941 — 2: 3.
132. Visibilidade do seio cavernoso — (Comunicação à Academia das Ciências de Lisboa, em 15 de Maio de 1941) — *Memórias da Academia das Ciências de Lisboa* — 1941 — 3: 403.
133. Circulação cerebral intermitente — *Imprensa Médica* — 1942 — 3: 65.
134. Angioma venoso do corp estriado. Sindroma parkinsónico lateralizado — (Comunicação à Academia das Ciências de Lisboa em 19 de Fevereiro de 1942) — *Imprensa Médica* — 1942 — no 4.
135. Diferenças de opacidades nos aneurismas cerebrais — *Lisboa Médica* — 1942 — 19: 123 — Separata de 8 pp.
136. Projecção em arteriografia lateral, de circulação anormal da carótida externa sobre a circulação cerebral — *Lisboa Médica* — 1942 — 19: 63.

137. Sobre a identificaçãa angiográfico das artérias e veias do cérebro — *Folia Anatomica Universitatis Conimbrigenis* — 1942 — 17: 1 — Separata de 9 pp.
138. Aspectos angiográficos dos glioblastomas — Em colaboração com Lobo Antunes — *Imprensa Médica* — 20: 165 — Separata de 11 pp.
139. Diagnostique angiographique des méningiomes de l'arête sphéniodale — *Schweizerische Medizinische Wochenschrift* — 1943 — 39: 51 — Separata de 12 pp.
140. Diagnóstico angiográfico dum angioma arterio-venoso cerebral com aneurisma intercalar — (Comunicação à Academia das Ciências de Lisboa em 4 de Março de 1943) — Memórias da Academia das Ciências de Lisboa — 1944: 4 — Separata de 2 pp.
141. Alterações da ampola e veias de Galeno nas dilatações ventriculares —Em colaboração com Lidia Manso Preto —*Lisboa Médica* — 1944 — 21: 1 — Separata de 9 pp.
142. A angiografia cerebral no diagnóstico das espécies tumorais — (Comunicação à Academia das Ciências de Lisboa em 17 de Fevereiro de 1944) — *Memórias da Academia das Ciências de Lisboa* — 1945 — 4: 3 — Separata de 7 pp.
143. Angiome de l'angle ponto-cérébelleux — Em colaboração com Abel Cancela de Abreu e Lobo Antunes — *Praxis* — 1944 — no 9 — Separata de 11 pp.
144. Capillaires du cerveau et de la tête. Déductions angiographies — Volume de homenagem ao Prof. A. Celestino da Costa — 1944 — *Amatus Lusitanus* — 1944 — 3: 506.
145. Novo aspecto angiográfico dos tumores da hipófise — Em colaboração com Joaquim Imaginário e Cruz e Silva — *Imprensa Médica* — 1944 — no 1 — Separata de 8 pp.
146. Os raios Roentgen na Neurologia — Conferéncia realizada na Sociedade de Ciências Médicas em 10 de Abril de 1945 — *Amatus Lusitanus* — 1945 — 4: 373 — Conferências — 1945 — 1: 68
147. Aspecto anormal da circulação do seio longitudinal inferior devido a compressão tumoral — (Comunicação à Academia das Ciências de Lisboa em 29 de Junho de 1944) — *Memórias da Academia das Ciências de Lisboa* — 1947 — 5 — Separata de 4 pp.
148. Thrombosis of the internal carotid and its branches — Presented to the Meeting of Society of British Neurological Surgeons — Monografia de 30 pp. illustrada com 12 figuras — *A Medicina Contemporânea* — 1947 — no 4 — Separata de 21 pp.

149. Trombose da carótida interna de etiologia traumática — (Comunicação à Classe de Ciências da Academia das Ciências de Lisboa em 5 de Julho de 1945) — *Memórias da Academia das Ciências de Lisboa* — 1948 — 5: 3 — Separata de 11 pp.

150. Contribuição da Escola Portuguesa para o futuro da Neurocirurgia — Oração pronunciada em francês pelo Prof. Almeida Lima, na sessão de abertura das "Giornate Mediche Internazionali" de Verona, em 20 de Julho de 1950, por delegação do Prof. Egas Moniz — Conferências — 1952 — 5: 8 — (Contém a fotografia da Medalha comemorativa das Jornadas, com a efigie do Prof. Egas Moniz).

151. Angioma arterio-venoso do cérebro — *A Medicina Contemporânea* — 1951 — no 6 — Separata de 10 pp.

152. Séméiologie angiographique des anévrismes, varices et angiomes du cerveau — Em colaboração com Miller Guerra — *Rapports du Véme Congrés Neurologique Internatcional* — 1953 — 3: 65.

153. Trombose da carótida interna. Visibilidade dos vasos da fossa posterior — (Comunicação à Classe de Ciências da Academia em 19 de Março de 1953) — Memórias da Acádemia das Ciências de Lisboa — 1953 —6 — *A Medicina Contemporânea* — 1953 — no 4 — Separata de 7 pp.

154. Subsidios para a história da angiografia — *Anais Azevedos* — 1955 — 7 — Separata de 21 pp.

PIONEERS IN RADIOLOGY — REYNALDO DOS SANTOS

1. A arteriografia dos membros — com Augusto Lamas e J. Pereira Caldas — *Medicina Contemporânea* — 1929.
2. Arteriografia da aorta e dos vasos abdominais — com Augusto Lamas e J. Pereira Caldas — *Medicina Contemporânea* — 1929.
3. L'artériographie des membres, de l'aorte et de ses branches abdominales — com Augusto Lamas e J. Pereira Caldas — *Bulletins et Mémoires de la Société Nationale de Chirurgie* — 1929.
4. L'artériographie de l'abdomen et des membres et les horizons de la voie artérielle — Conférence du 22 Mars 1929 à la Clinique Chirurgicale du Prof. Leriche à l'Université de Strasbourg — *Medicina Contemporânea* — 1929.
5. Abdominopelvine arteriographie (aortographie) — Verhandlungen der deutschen Röntgen-Gesellschaft — 1931.
6. Les récents progrès dans la tecnique de l'artériographie de l'aorte abdominale — com Augusto Lamas e J. Pereira Caldas — *Presse Médicale* — No. 31 — 1931.
7. Les dérivés du thorium dans l'artériographie des membres — com J. Pereira Caldas — *Medicina Contemporânea* — 1931.
8. Reflexões sobre certos problemas fisio-patológicos de circulação e dos ógãos e interpretaçao da toxicade de certos medicamentos à luz da arteriografia — Discurso inaugural do ano académico da Sociedade das Ciências Médicas de Lisboa, em 12 de Dezembro de 1931.
9. Estudos funcionais de arteriografia — com Augusto Lamas e J. Pereira Caldas — *Medicina Contemporânea* — Março 1932.
10. Novo caso de arteriografia de sarcoma do baço — *Revista Médico-Farmacêutica* — 1932.
11. L'artériographie des membres — com Augusto Lamas e J. Pereira Caldas — *Bulletins et Mémoires de la Société Nationale de Chirurgie* — 1932.
12. L'arteriographie en Sirie — *Bulletins of Mémoires de la Société Nationale de Chirurgie* — 1932.
13. Quisto hidático para-renal, diagnosticado pela aortografia — com Fernando Lacerda — *Medicina Contemporânea* — 1933.
14. - Pyélographie descendante — *Medicina Contemporânea* — 1933.
15. Nouvelles applications cliniques de l'aortographie à quelques problèmes de chirurgie rénale — Communication au Congrés d'Urologie, Paris, Octobre, 1933.

16. L'aortographie dans les tumeurs rénales et para-rénales — Communication au Congrès de l'Association Française d'urologie, Octobre, 1933 — *Lisboa Médica* — 1933 — *Archives des maladies des reins et des organes génito-urinaires* — 1934.
17. L'artériographie dans les néoplasies des os et des parties molles — *Bulletins et Mémoires de la Société National de Chirurgie* — 1934.
18. L'opération de Mattas à la lumiére de l'artériographie — *Bulletins et Mémoires de la Société Nationale de Chirurgie* — 1934.
19. As gangrenas dos membros — *Medicina* — 1934.
20. L'artériographie dans le diagnostic des tumeurs osseuses — *Mémoires de l'Académie de Chirurgie* — 1936.
21. Les indications de la chirurgie du sympathique dans les artérites — A propos de la discussion de la "Gangliectomie lombaire" au Congrès du Caire — *Lisboa Médica* — 1936.
22. Les injections intra-artérielles dans les infections hématogénes du rein — *Congrès de Vienne* — *Lisboa Médica* — 1936.
23. A via carotidiana no tratamento das meningites — *Medicina Contemporânea* — 1937.
24. As injecções intra-arteriais nas infecções gravis dos membros — *Medicina Contemporânea* — 1937.
25. Syndrome causalgique après phlébite de la veine axillaire — Résection du ganglion étoilé — *Presse Médicale,* 30 — 1937.
26. Les embolies artèrielles des membres — *Medicina Contemporânea* — 1937.
27. A aortografia nas doenças cirúrgicas do baço — com António Carneiro de Moura — *Medicina Contemporânea* — 1937.
28. Traitement des phlébites et de leurs séquelles —*Medicina Contemporânea* — 1937.
29. Tecnique de l'aortographie — *Journal International de Chirurgie* — 1937.
30. La voie artérielle dans la séméiologie et la thérapeutique — *Schémas* — no. 10 — Maio 1939.
31. Os aneurismas arteriais dos membros — *Amatus Lusitanus* — Vol. I — P. 233 — 1942.
32. Lipo mio-angioma parcialmente sarcomatoso bilateral dos rins (arteriografia) com doença quistica dos pulmões — 1942.

33. L'artériographie — *Rapport au Congrès de la Société Internationale de Chirurgie* — Londres — 1947.
34. L'artériographie des membres et de l'aorte abdominal — (Livro publicado em francês) *Masson* — Paris 1931.

PIONEERS IN RADIOLOGY — LOPO de CARVALHO

1. Visualizačão aos Raios X, dos vasos pulmonares, obtida por injecção de liquido opaco na auricula direita — *Acad. Ciências de Lisboa* — III — 1931.
2. Sur la sensibilité des veines du cou et de l'oreillette droite — *Soc. Biol.* CVII — 1931.
3. La circulation veineuse du cou et la décharge veineuse de l'encéphale — *Soc. Biol.* CVII — 1931.
4. La visibilité des vaisseaux pulmonaires aux rayons X par injection, dans l'oreillette droite, de fortes solutions d'iodure de sodium. — *Acad. Med. Paris* — 1931.
5. Le sondage des veines et la pression dans les troncs veineux de l'Homme — *Soc. Biol.* CVII— 1931.
6. Angiopneumographie — *Presse Médical* — 53 — 1931.
7. Aus dem Gebiet der Angiopneumographie. — *Beit Klin. Tub.* — 79 — 1931.
8. L'Angiopneumographie et son application dans la Tuberculose pulmonaire — *Presse Médicale* — 56 — 1932.
9. La visibilité des vaisseaux pulmonaires (Angiopneumographie) — *J. Rad. Elect.* — 10 — 1932.
10. Die Angiopneumographie — *Beit. Klin. Tub.* — 5 — 1932.
11. A visibilidade dos vasos pulmonares (Angiopneumography) — *Lisboa Médica* — 1932.
12. The visibility of the pulmonary vessels (Angiopneumography) — *Act. Rad.* — 5 — 1933.
13. Une méthode pour l'étude de l'anatomie du Poumon — *Fol. Anat.* — 16 — 1933.
14. Imagens arteriais do hilo e topografia arterial do pulmão — *Lisboa Mé*dica — 1934.
15. Topographie artérielle du poumon — *Presse Médicale* — 102 — 1934.
16. O modo d'acção do pneumotórax artificial — *Lisboa Méd.* — 1934.
17. Mode d'action du pneumothorax — *Rev. Tub.* — 5 — 1935.
18. Les aspects radiologiques du hile et leur interpretation — *Union Int. Tub.* — 1936.
19. Les aspects radiologiques du hile pulmonaire et leur interprétation (Discussion Générale) — *Union Int. Tub.* — 1937.
20. Angiopneumography — *Cong. Lourenço Marques* — 1938.
21. Angiopneumografia. Sua importância para a interpretaçao das Radiografias Torácicas — *Imp. Med.* — 1938.

22. L'Angiopneumographie et l'Interprétation des Radiographies thoraciques — *Schemas* — 10 — 1939.
23. Der Lungenkreislauf unter patologischen Umständen — *Beit. Klin. Tub.* — 95 — 1940.
24. Angiopneumografia. Sua importância para o estudo das alteraçöes da circulação pulmonar — *Bol. Soc. Rad.* — III — 1940.
25. Imagens arterials do hilo — *Lições de Tisiologia* — 1942.
26. Angiopneumografia — *Lições de Tisiologia* — 1942.
27. A velocidade da circulação pulmonar. — *Acad. Ciências Lisboa* — V — 1947.
28. La Velocidad de la Circulacion pulmonar — *Rev. Clinica Esp.* — 4 — 1947.
29. La Vitesse de la Circulation pulmonaire — *Bul Soc. Med. Hôp.* — 7 — 1948.
30. A velocidade de circulação pulmonar — *Coimbra Médica* — 4 — 1948.
31. La vitesse de la circulation pulmonaire — *Presse Medicale* — 57 — 1948.
32. L'Angiopneumographie — Sa contribution à l'interprétation des radiographies du thorax et son importance pour l'étude de la circulation pulmonaire — *Acta Tub.* — 3 — 1948.
33. Nouvelles applications des principes de la Chymographie — *Bruxelles Méd.* — 1948.
34. Die Röntgenkymographie bei der Untersuchung des Lungenkreislauf — *Rad. Clin.* — XVIII — 1949.
35. Localização apical da Tuberculose pulmonar no adulto — *Acad. Ciências Lisboa* — 1949.
36. Estudo quimográfico de pequena circulação — *Rad. Canc.* — 1949.
37. Novas aplicações da Quimografia — *Clin. Tis.* — 13 — 1949.
38. Nova técnica par exames angiocardiopneumográficos — *An. Azevedo* — 2 — 1949.
39. Angiocardiopneumography — *Diseases of the Chest* — 1950.
40. Une technique nouvelle pour les examens angiocardiopneumographiques — *Bul. Soc. Méd. Hôp.* — 25 — 1950.
41. Les antibiotiques associés ou non au pneumothorax et la vascularisation du poumon — *Union Int. Tun.* — 1950.
42. L'enregistrement radiographique de la circulation capillaire du poumon — *Bul. Acad. Méd.* — 15 — 1951.

43. La circulation pulmonaire en différentes situations pathologiques (Recherches angiopneumographiques) — *Rev. Tub.* — 6 — 1951.
44. Uma nova técnica para os exames angiopneumográficos — *Cli. Hig. e Hidro.* — 1 — 1951.
45. A circulacão pulmonar em diversas situações patológicas. Investigações angiopneumográficas — *Méd. Contemp.* — 5 — 1951.
46. Contribuição da angiopneumografia para a apreciação das propriedades farmacodinâmicas de alguns medicamentos. — *Med. Contemp.* — 9 — 1952.
47. Novas perspectivas da Angiocardiopneumografia — *O Médico* — 70 — 1953.
48. Nuevas perspectivas de la angio-cardio pneumografia— 5a — *Jorn. Arg. Cir. Tor.* — 1953.
49. Angiopneumography in the Study of the Pharmacodynamic Properties of certain drugs — *Diseases of the Chest.* — 2 — 1954.
50. Circulation bronchique et pulmonaire — Leur interdépendance — *Les Bronches* — VI — 1956.
51. Die Angiopneumographie — *Ihre Geschicte* — 1957.
52. The Angiocardiopneumography — General considerations — Chapter of the Book — *Roentgenology of the Chest* — 1957.
53. Hémoptysies et Anastomoses artério-veineuses — *Paris* — 1957.
54. Les hémoptysies bronco-pulmonaires — *Les Bronches* — VIII — 1958.
55. Anastomoses artério-veineuses — *Journal Français de Médecine et Chirurgie Thoraciques* — XII — 1958.
56. As anastomoses artério-venosas da rede vascular do pulmão — *Jornal da Sociedade das Ciências Médicas de Lisboa* — 1959.

PIONEER IN RADIOLOGY — HERNANI MONTEIRO

1. A regulação nervosa dos vasos. Subsidios para o estudo da inervação do sistema linfático. — *sep. A Medicina Contemporânea* — no. 24, Ano LX, 1942.

2. L'état actuel; de la lymphangiographie chez le vivant — *Trabalhos de Anatomia* — 1934-1935. (Em colaboração com Alvaro Rodrigues e Sousa Pereira).

3. Etudes sur l'Anatomo-Physiologie du système lymphatique — I — Action du sympatique sur le courant de la lymphe dans le canal thoracique — *Societé Portugais de Biologie* — Tome III, No. 19 — *Arq. dos Trabalhos da Faculdade de Medicina do Porto* — 1947 — II — Action de l'adrenaline, de l'acetylcholine, de l'histamine et de la pituitrine sur le courant de la lymphe du canal thoracique — *Sociéte Portugaise de Biologie* — Tome VIII, 1947. — III — Action du Sympathique sur les parois des vaisseaux lymphatiques — *Societé Portugaise de Biologie* — Tome X. 1950. (Em colaboração com Silva Pinto).

4. Visibilidade do sistema linfático no vivo — *Portugal Médico* — XXIII, 5, 195-208, 1934.

5. Métodos do estudo do sistema linfático no vivo — *Boletim da Sociedade Portugesa de Radiologia Médica* — 4, 2, 3-34, 1941. — La voie lymphatique — *Extrait de Schemas* — no. 10, Mai 1939. (Em colaboração com Alvaro Rodrigues, Sousa Pereira e Roberto Carvalho).

7. Acção das simpaticectomias e das infiltrações novocainicas do simpatico sobre o sistema linfático — *Sep. da Imprensa Médica* — Ano. VII, no. 11, 1941. (Em colaboração com Alvaro Rodrigues, Roberto Carvalho e Sousa Pereira).

8. La méthode radiographique de mise en évidence des lymphatiques chez le vivant et ses applications — *Journal International de Chirurgie* Bruxelles, II, 6, 655-670, 1937. (Em colaboração com Roberto Carvalho, Alvaro Rodrigues e Sousa Pereira).

9. Investigações sobre a fisiopatologia neurolinfática — *Portugal Médico* — XLII, 445-468, 1958. (Em colaboração com A. Rodrigues. A. Sousa Pereira e Silva Pinto).

10. Para a história do estudo do sistema linfático no vivo — *Boletim de la Universidad de Santiago* — 1933. (Em colaboração com Alvaro Rodrigues, Robert Carvalho e Sousa Pereira).

11. Méthodes de demonstration du Système Lymphatique chez le vivant — *Extrait des C.R. de l'Association des Anatomistes* — XLIIIe. Réunion. Lisbonne, 26-29 Mars 1957. (Em colaboração

com Alvaro Rodgrigues, A. Tavares e Albano Ramos).
12. Sistema linfático. Contribuição do centro de estudo de medicina experimental para o conhecimento da sua anatomofisiologia — *Gazeta Médica Portuguesa* — 741-748, 1954. (Em colaboração com M. SIlva Pinto e A. Sampaio Tavares).
13. Circulação linfática e estase venosa — *Portugal Médico* — XLIII, 1, 1-7, 1959. (Em colaboração com A. S. Tavares).
14. La lymphangeographie chez le vivant (méthodes, résultats et applications) — *Bruxelles-Médical* — nos. 7 e 8 — Dezembro de 1938.
15. Técnica de injecção de linfáticos no animal vivo — *Medicina* — Madrid — Dezembro — 1946.

PIONEERS IN RADIOLOGY — JOAO CID DOS SANTOS

1. Aspects normaux de l'artériographie des membres et de l'aorte abdominale sur le vivant — com Reynaldo dos Santos — *Comptes-rendus de la XXVIIIéme. Réunion de l'Association des Anatomistes* — Lisbonne — 1933.
2. A flebografia — *Medicina Contemporânea* — 1937.
3. La transfusion de sang par voie aortique. Valeur générale de cette voie pour l'introduction de médicaments dans le sang — *Medicina Contemporânea* — 1937.
4. Études sur l'artériographie normale du chien — com D. Benoliel, O. Fragoso e N. Nunes — *Medicina Contemporânea* — 1937.
5. Spasme veineux du bras aprés injection intra-artérielle. Action de l'infiltration du ganglion étoilé. Contrôle phlébographie avant et après l'infiltration — *Rev. de Chir.* — no. 4 — Abril 1938.
6. Revisão dos problemas fisio-patológicos e terapêuticos das embolias das extremidades á luz do factor vasomotor — *Medicina Contemporânea* — 1938.
7. La phlébographie directe. Conception. Technique. Premiers résultats — *Journal International de Chirurgie* — 1938.
8. Embolia da origem da artéria úmeral. Embolectomia. Cura. Importância do espasmo gerado ao nível da sutura na determinação da trombose pós-operatória e melos de a combater — *Amatus Lusitanus* — 1943.
9. Patologia geral das isquémias dos membros. Ensaio baseado no seu aspecto clinico. (Tese de doutoramento) — *Livraria Luso-Espanhola* — 1944.
10. Aneurisma da origem da femural. Aortografia. Operação de Mattas com compressão da aorta e autrotransfusão. Cura — *Amatus Lusitanus* — 1944.
11. Sobre a embolectomia — *Lisboa Médica* — 1944.
12. Embolectomia da aorta terminal — *Amatus Lusitanus* — 1944.
13. Embolia dos membros — Lições de patologia cirúrgica geral — por Reynaldo dos Santos e seus colaboradores — *Livraria Luso-Espanhola* — 1946.
14. Sobre a embolectomia das artérias dos membros. Bases para uma nova orientação do problema — *Amatus Lusitanus* — 1948.
15. Sur la désobstruction des thromboses artérielles anciennes (Rapport de M. R. Leriche) — *Bulletins et Mém. de l'Académie de Chirurgie* — P. 409 — 1947.
16. Sur quelques vérités premières oubliées ou méconnues de l'anatomophysiologie normale et pathologique du système veineux. Leur application à la pathologie et à la pathologie et à

la thérapeutique — Conférence aux Journées Cardiologiques Internationales — Paris — 1947. *Amatus Lusitanus* — 1948.
17. The diagnosis and treatment of vascular obstruction — Hunterian lecture for the annual meeting of the Hunterian Society — 1948 — *Gazeta Médica* — 1948.
18. L'Angiographie rénale — Xéme. Congrès de la Société Internationale d'Urologie — Atenas — 1955.
19. Arteriography of the extremities in peripheral vascular diseases — 3o. Congresso Mundial de Cardiologia — Bruxelas — 1958.
20. An Introduction to Phlebography of the Lower Limbs — 9o. Congresso da Sociedade Europeia de Cirurgia Cardio-Vascular — Barcelona — 1960.
21. Le traitement général des ischémies aiguës — 11o. Congresso da Sociedade Europeia de Cirurgia Cardio-Vascular — Estocolmo — Julho — 1962.
22. Late results of reconstructive arterial surgery — Restoration — Disobliteration — Replacement with the establishment of some operative principles — 6o. Congresso da Sociedade Internacional de Cardiologia — Roma — 1963.
23. Un temps essentiel de l'endartériectomie: le dépassement du bord de l'endartère distale (overpass) — *Mémoires de l'Académie de Chirurgie* — T. 90 — P. 683 — 1964.

PIONEERS IN RADIOLOGY — SOUSA PEREIRA

1. O estudo flebográfico do sistema porta (colab. Melo Adrião e dr Lino Rodgrigues) — *Academia das Ciências de Lisboa*, 5 — 1951.
2. La méthode phlébografique dans l'étude des troubles de la circulation du système porte — *I Cong. Mondial de Cardiologie.*
3. 1950 e *Lyon Chirurgical*, 46, 3 — 1951.
4. Étude phlébographique et éssais thérapeutiques dans la thrombose des veines du système portal (col. profs. J. Azevedo Maia e Melo Adrião e drs. Lino Rodrigues e Aguiar Nogueira) — *1ème Cong. de la Soc. Intern. de Chirurgie*, 1951.
5. Thrombose aigüle de la veine porte et de ses branches — *Congresso Europeu de gasteroenterologia.* Julho de 1954.

INDEX

GPSR Compliance

The European Union's (EU) General Product Safety Regulation (GPSR) is a set of rules that requires consumer products to be safe and our obligations to ensure this.

If you have any concerns about our products, you can contact us on ProductSafety@springernature.com

In case Publisher is established outside the EU, the EU authorized representative is:

Springer Nature Customer Service Center GmbH
Europaplatz 3
69115 Heidelberg, Germany

Batch number: 10584444

Printed by Printforce, the Netherlands